Quality Improvement in Nursing

Sara Miller McCune founded SAGE Publishing in 1965 to support the dissemination of usable knowledge and educate a global community. SAGE publishes more than 1000 journals and over 800 new books each year, spanning a wide range of subject areas. Our growing selection of library products includes archives, data, case studies and video. SAGE remains majority owned by our founder and after her lifetime will become owned by a charitable trust that secures the company's continued independence.

Los Angeles | London | New Delhi | Singapore | Washington DC | Melbourne

Quality Improvement in Nursing

Edited by
Gillian Janes
Catherine Delves-Yates

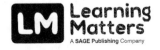
Learning Matters
A SAGE Publishing Company

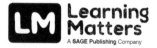

Learning Matters
A SAGE Publishing Company
1 Oliver's Yard
55 City Road
London EC1Y 1SP

SAGE Publications Inc.
2455 Teller Road
Thousand Oaks, California 91320

SAGE Publications India Pvt Ltd
B 1/I 1 Mohan Cooperative Industrial Area
Mathura Road
New Delhi 110 044

SAGE Publications Asia-Pacific Pte Ltd
3 Church Street
#10-04 Samsung Hub
Singapore 049483

Editors: Laura Walmsley
Development editor: Cassie Fox
Senior project editor: Chris Marke
Project management: River Editorial
Marketing manager: Ruslana Khatagova
Cover design: Sheila Tong
Typeset by: C&M Digitals (P) Ltd, Chennai, India

Library of Congress Control Number: 2022943221

British Library Cataloguing in Publication Data

A catalogue record for this book is available from the British Library

ISBN 978-1-5297-6896-1
ISBN 978-1-5297-6897-8 (pbk)

Contents

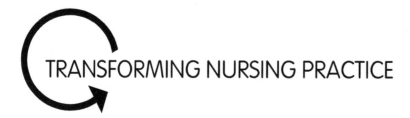

TRANSFORMING NURSING PRACTICE

Transforming Nursing Practice is a series tailor made for pre-registration student nurses. Each book in the series is:

- Affordable
- Full of active learning features
- Mapped to the NMC Standards of proficiency for registered nurses
- Focused on applying theory to practice

Each book addresses a core topic and they have been carefully developed to be simple to use, quick to read and written in clear language.

An invaluable series of books that explicitly relates to the NMC standards. Each book covers a different topic that students need to explore in order to develop into a qualified nurse... I would recommend this series to all Pre-Registered nursing students whatever their field or year of study.

LINDA ROBSON,
Senior Lecturer at Edge Hill University

Many titles in the series are on our recommended reading list and for good reason - the content is up to date and easy to read. These are the books that actually get used beyond training and into your nursing career.

EMMA LYDON,
Adult Student Nursing

ABOUT THE SERIES EDITORS

DR MOOI STANDING is an Independent Nursing Consultant (UK and International) and is responsible for the core knowledge, adult nursing and personal and professional learning skills titles. She is an experienced NMC Quality Assurance Reviewer of educational programmes and a Professional Regulator Panellist on the NMC Practice Committee. Mooi is also Board member of Special Olympics Malaysia, enabling people with intellectual disabilities to participate in sports and athletics nationally and internationally.

DR SANDRA WALKER is a Clinical Academic in Mental Health working between Southern Health Trust and the University of Southampton and responsible for the mental health nursing titles. She is a Qualified Mental Health Nurse with a wide range of clinical experience spanning more than 25 years.

BESTSELLING TEXTBOOKS

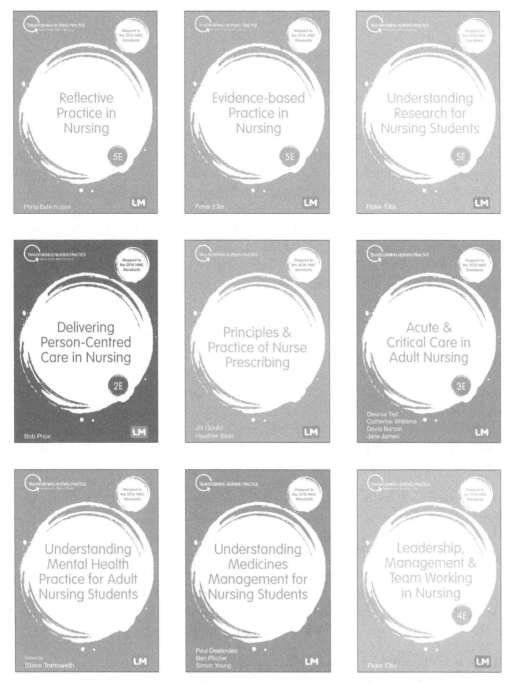

You can find a full list of textbooks in the *Transforming Nursing Practice* series at
https://uk.sagepub.com/TNP-series

About the authors

Claire Brockwell is Lecturer in Nursing Sciences at the University of East Anglia. Claire was a 'Why?' child and maintaining this approach in adulthood enabled her to enquire into, seek to understand and help resolve short-term and longer-term problems in diverse environments including large-scale leadership, finance and project management. Nurturing innovation skills in others and overlaying that with an understanding of the importance of governance and strategy allowed Claire to co-ordinate a review board for projects in business skills that, following her nursing degree, Claire transferred to managing an NHS research team. Claire's doctoral study was based on collaboratively developing and testing an intervention relating to empowering self-management in chronic disease. In her current role Claire loves to kindle the flame of curiosity and the ability to manage change for patient benefit in future health and social care professionals.

Michelle Croston is an Associate Professor at the University of Nottingham. She has a clinical background in HIV care working at national and international level to improve outcomes for people living with HIV. She holds a fellowship with the European Society of Person Centered Healthcare (ESPCH). Michelle has extensive postgraduate qualifications in mental health and psychological trauma, and alongside her academic role she is a qualified Crisis Counsellor for a Mental Health charity that specialises in working with healthcare workers. Michelle is passionate about developing teaching and learning strategies to prevent compassion fatigue and secondary trauma.

Catherine Delves-Yates is an experienced nurse and a Lecturer at the University of East Anglia. After starting her nursing career at the Nightingale School London, she has worked clinically in adult and paediatric critical care in the UK and has nursed and taught in America, Africa and Nepal. Her passion is to ensure all nurses have the knowledge, skills and professionalism to deliver effective compassionate care to each of their patients. Catherine is an Honorary Lecturer in Universities in Cameroon and Nepal. Currently she is researching whether nursing students' views of health and illness alter during their pre-registration nursing programme.

Jill Foley is a registered adult nurse with extensive leadership, curriculum development and teaching experience. She has led the development of pre-registration nursing programmes at undergraduate and MSc level and, as a principal lecturer, supported pre- and post-registration course teams in the design, implementation and evaluation of university and practice-based programmes. Jill held consultancy roles during the development of the NMC (2010) Standards for pre-registration nursing education and the Standards framework for nursing and midwifery education (NMC 2018). She has also worked as an NMC Quality Assurance Visitor for nursing and nursing associate programmes. She is committed to championing and fostering excellence in nursing practice through education, innovation and research. Quality improvement, co-production, leadership, and developing personal capability to deliver compassionate, high-quality nursing care has been a focus of her work.

Daniel Heggie is an adult nurse who is currently working as a Clinical Research Team Leader on a national Cancer Research trial. His passion for quality improvement came when he began to ask the question 'Why do we get students to complete all this research and let it not be implemented?' This led to him working with colleagues to construct an annual regional improvement conference. He enjoys cooking (but mainly eating) and going on long walks on the beach with his dog and his partner.

Gillian Janes is an experienced nurse, educator and researcher. She is an Associate Clinical Fellow at Manchester Metropolitan University and Honorary Associate Professor, Macquarie University, Sydney. She works nationally and internationally, enabling organisations to create the right system conditions for service improvement, and developing the workforce to ensure they have the personal, technical and strategic knowledge and skills to enable them to use Improvement Science to aid patient safety and healthcare quality. Gillian's PhD used silences research to improve services based on patient experience. She is a National Institute for Health Research (NIHR) Academy Member; NHS Q Community Founding Cohort member and Trustee of the Clinical Human Factors Group.

Mark Morson is a Clinical Educator and Bank Staff Nurse at the Norfolk and Norwich University Hospital. In his Clinical Educator role, he specialises in the support of pre-registered student nurses in practice. Mark is also a Clinical Skills Lecturer in the School of Health Sciences at the University of East Anglia where he specialises in teaching pre-registered student nurses clinical skills as preparation for practice. Mark has a particular passion for supporting student-led quality improvement initiatives and recognises their value to modern health services. In particular, Mark has been impressed by the quality and inventiveness of initiatives produced by final year student nurses as part of their capstone projects.

Nickey Rooke is an Associate Professor in the School of Health Sciences at the University of East Anglia. Her nursing career began over 30 years ago and, since qualifying, Nickey has worked predominantly in Older People's Medicine and the community where she worked as a District Nursing Sister for several years before moving into Higher Education. Nickey is involved in teaching across a variety of nursing programmes including nursing apprenticeships, undergraduate, postgraduate and post-registration programmes, and is currently Course Director for MSc Adult Nursing. She was awarded a PhD in Nursing Studies from the University of Essex in 2018, and her interests include patient and public involvement in practice assessment, quality improvement, community nursing, leadership and health education.

Editors' acknowledgements

We would like to express our gratitude to: all the people accessing care and their families, colleagues and students who have provided us with the experience and experiences needed to develop this book. Jill Foley for her knowledge, insight and attention to detail in compiling the mapping to the NMC proficiencies. Martin-Delves-Yates for turning our confused scribblings into clear and simple line drawings. All the contributors who, despite a worldwide pandemic and other unexpected major life events, found the time to draft, rewrite, and craft their chapters. Laura Walmsley at Sage for having the foresight to commission the book in the first place. And finally, Marty and the 'family Janes' plus Martin and Florence Delves-Yates for their support, encouragement and acceptance that they would be cooking supper, again!

Introduction

Gillian Janes and Catherine Delves-Yates

Quality improvement (QI) is a cornerstone of modern healthcare. Unsurprisingly, healthcare organisations expect their staff not just to be safe and effective nurses but also to be able to work with service users, carers and colleagues to improve the work they do, and the quality of care delivered. Achieving this is a complex process that requires healthcare practitioners to draw on theory and practice from a range of scientific disciplines. This book therefore draws together key information to guide you through every stage of the improvement process, enabling you to apply this knowledge in your own practice.

Who should read the book?

You should read this book if you are leading an improvement, either in theory or practice, perhaps for your final dissertation/major project; or if you aspire to be more formally involved in improving the quality and/or safety of healthcare more widely. The book is designed for pre-registration nursing students at any academic level but is also appropriate for students and staff from other healthcare disciplines studying this topic. In addition, quality improvement faculty who are seeking a tried and tested approach to teaching quality improvement and useful resources to support student learning on this topic will find the book equally relevant. UK healthcare practice is the main focus; however, quality improvement is an international discipline, therefore resources are also drawn from elsewhere.

Why read the book?

It will help you develop an in-depth understanding of your quality improvement role, an improvement mind-set and the ability to apply the principles of Improvement Science in your everyday practice. The aim is to de-mystify the improvement that staff often do intuitively, while developing an awareness of how this can be **aligned** with the formal, **systematic** approach to Improvement Science and the academic literature.

As a core part of the nursing role, developing and demonstrating improvement expertise will enhance your employability. This is because quality improvement is not only an important means of achieving better health outcomes and the experience of people accessing services as part of values-based practice, but it can also be used to enhance staff retention, experience and wellbeing. This in turn influences the quality and safety of care.

An initial, more detailed discussion of the relevance of quality improvement for nurses and nursing is provided in Chapter 1, then built on throughout the book. As is consistent with this type of introductory textbook, core concepts will be developed in-depth, supplemented by an initial discussion and signposting to further resources and specific specialist expertise where appropriate, as for example with the Human Factors material in Chapter 2.

How is the book structured?

The book is in three main parts: each part opens with the experience of an individual whose goals and characteristics represent the needs of a larger group that the chapters in that part of the book relate to. The book also encourages you to identify and apply the complementary knowledge and skills you already have or are developing to your quality improvement practice. Examples of this transferable expertise include evidence-informed practice, research, patient safety, leadership and professional accountability. Where relevant, you will also be directed to other titles in the TNP series, e.g. leadership or patient safety, to support your learning in specific areas.

Part 1: Establishing the context

Chapter 1 'What is quality improvement and why is it important?' explores how QI has evolved to be recognised as a fundamentally important aspect of the role of a healthcare professional today and how nurses can contribute to enhancing the quality of care for service users.

Chapter 2 'Understanding the principles of quality improvement and your own contribution' introduces a range of improvement principles, commonly used methods and tools and their application in practice. This chapter also enables you to explore and develop the personal leadership qualities and skills needed to exercise professional citizenship for healthcare improvement.

Part 2: Developing skills for quality improvement

Chapter 3 'Leading change and working with others' explores change theory and the principles of leading change. A range of tools is introduced to support partnership working and collaborative improvement in practice and activities are provided to enable you to apply these within the context of your role.

Chapter 4 'Identifying and justifying the need for service improvement' introduces some key considerations and commonly used tools and draws on learning from previous chapters to enable you to identify and develop an evidence-based, contextualised and sustainable improvement idea of relevance to practice, focusing particularly on the application of Part 1 of the Model for Improvement (MFI).

Chapter 5 'Planning and implementing improvement' demonstrates how it is possible to apply the entire MFI, including some of the methods, tools and approaches highlighted in preceding chapters to develop a systematic and implementable quality improvement. An integral aspect of this is the persistent focus upon the importance of including stakeholders at every stage.

Chapter 6 'Evaluating and sustaining improvement' establishes evaluation as a foundational aspect of any improvement activity and explores the role it plays in sustaining change. The chapter introduces and illustrates the application of relevant models and frameworks along with activities to enable you to explore how you might evaluate and sustain your improvement in practice.

Part 3: Moving forward

Chapter 7 'Quality improvement: the next decade' explores current progress and identifies some future priorities for healthcare improvement. It does this within the context of what the profession and individual practitioners can contribute to the improvement agenda moving forward and how to achieve this, working in partnership with service users and the public as part of a multidisciplinary team.

Chapter 8 'Quality improvement and you: the future' provides an opportunity to review how your quality improvement expertise has developed and plan some practical next steps to further enhance this as you progress to the next stage in your career. This chapter adopts a dual focus on how to further develop the technical components of your improvement knowledge and skills as well as the broader leadership and change agent capabilities needed to successfully apply these.

General points
Terminology

While different terminology may be used in particular healthcare settings, the following terms will be used throughout the book. These have been chosen to align with Nursing and Midwifery Council (NMC) terminology, promote a person-centred, inclusive approach and maximise clarity/shared understanding, i.e.:

- people, service users or people accessing services – rather than patients;
- carers – includes carers and significant others;

- student nurses or nursing students – this may equally be relevant for students of other healthcare disciplines;
- registered nurses or healthcare staff rather than 'qualified staff'.

Though terms such as 'your project' may be used in the text to encourage personal ownership and emphasise your lead role in a particular improvement initiative, we encourage you to interpret its use with care as it can be unhelpful in communicating the shared ownership and engagement of others that is required for any sustained improvement. The importance of interprofessional practice and the crucial role of relevant **stakeholders** in any improvement activity is emphasised throughout because improvement is a person-centred activity that must often be enacted through interprofessional collaboration to be successful (Montgomery et al, 2020). This involves striking a balance between taking individual and enabling shared responsibility based on an awareness of how language facilitates or hinders this delicate balance.

NMC proficiencies

The content of this book is aligned with, though not limited to, the requirements of *Future Nurse: Standards of Proficiency for Registered Nurses* (NMC, 2018a). These require nurses to be able to undertake quality improvement within the context of their own practice. The proficiencies are grouped under seven platforms as shown in Box I.1, and together with the two skills annexes reflect what newly registered nurses are expected to know and be capable of doing safely and proficiently as they embark on their career. The platforms are all interconnected; therefore, while the content of this book is of most relevance to platform six, it also supports aspects of platforms one, five and seven and the broader achievement of all seven. The main platforms and the proficiencies each chapter supports are listed at the start of each chapter.

Box I.1   Future Nurse: Standards for Proficiency for Registered Nurses Platforms

Platform 1: Being an accountable professional

Registered nurses act in the best interests of people, putting them first and providing nursing care that is person-centred, safe and compassionate. They act professionally at all times and use their knowledge and experience to make evidence-based decisions about care. They communicate effectively, are role models for others, and are accountable for their actions. Registered nurses continually reflect on their practice and keep abreast of new and emerging developments in nursing, health and care.

Platform 2: Promoting health and preventing ill health

Registered nurses play a key role in improving and maintaining the mental, physical and behavioural health and wellbeing of people, families, communities and populations. They support and enable people at all stages of life and in all care settings to make informed choices about how to manage health challenges to maximise their quality of life and improve health outcomes. They are actively involved in the prevention of and protection against disease and ill health and engage in public health, community development and global health agendas, and in the reduction of health inequalities.

Platform 3: Assessing needs and planning care

Registered nurses prioritise the needs of people when assessing and reviewing their mental, physical, cognitive, behavioural, social and spiritual needs. They use information obtained during assessments to identify the priorities and requirements for person-centred and evidence-based nursing interventions and support. They work in partnership with people to develop person-centred care plans that take into account their circumstances, characteristics and preferences.

Platform 4: Providing and evaluating care

Registered nurses take the lead in providing evidence-based, compassionate and safe nursing interventions. They ensure the care they provide and delegate is person-centred and of a consistently high standard. They support people of all ages in a range of care settings. They work in partnership with people, families and carers to evaluate whether care is effective and the goals of care have been met in line with their wishes, preferences and desired outcomes.

Platform 5: Leading and managing nursing care and working in teams

Registered nurses provide leadership by acting as role models for best practice in the delivery of nursing care. They are responsible for managing nursing care and are accountable for the appropriate delegation and supervision of care provided by others in the team including lay carers. They play an active and equal role in the interdisciplinary team, collaborating and communicating effectively with a range of colleagues.

Platform 6: Improving safety and quality of care

Registered nurses make a key contribution to the continuous monitoring and quality improvement of care and treatment to enhance health outcomes and people's experience of nursing and related care. They assess risks to safety or experience and take appropriate action to manage those, putting the best interests, needs and preferences of people first.

Platform 7: Co-ordinating care

Registered nurses play a leadership role in co-ordinating and managing the complex nursing and integrated care needs of people at any stage of their lives, across a range of organisations and settings. They contribute to processes of organisational change through an awareness of local and national policies.

Learning features

Each chapter contains brief case studies to help illustrate the topics covered in the book. Worked examples are provided throughout to demonstrate the application of the tools and concepts introduced, along with guided learning activities to enable you to apply these in your own practice.

Other features

The book is designed to enable you to develop your own quality improvement **glossary** of key terms by combining the short glossaries provided in each chapter, to which you are encouraged to add your own as you progress. Specific terms related to quality improvement are included in the glossary for the chapter in which they are first used. These are presented in bold in the text as shown by the word '**glossary**' earlier in this paragraph.

Glossary

Aligned: to correctly position an item in relation to something else
Glossary: a vocabulary or alphabetical list providing a brief explanation of newly introduced, uncommon, or specialised terms
Stakeholders: anyone who has a stake in a particular issue or the outcome
Systematic: methodical, organised, logical

Foundations chapter

Gillian Janes and Catherine Delves-Yates

NMC Future Nurse: Standards of Proficiency for Registered Nurses

This chapter will address the following platforms and proficiencies:

Platform 1: Being an accountable professional

1.2 understand and apply relevant legal, regulatory and governance requirements, policies and ethical frameworks, including any mandatory reporting duties, to all areas of practice, differentiating where appropriate between the devolved legislatures of the United Kingdom.

Platform 6: Improving safety and quality of care

6.4 demonstrate an understanding of the principles of improvement methodologies, participate in all stages of audit activity and identify appropriate quality improvement strategies.

Introduction

Facilitating improvement in practice is not a linear process and requires the integrated application of a range of theories and practical tools alongside the transferable knowledge and skills you are already mastering as part of the nursing programme. This chapter aims to put you on a sure footing for achieving this by enabling you to develop the fundamental knowledge and an outline of how to get the best out of the book; this includes an explanation of the conceptual model of healthcare improvement that we use to guide the content of the book and the adaptation of Langley et al's (2009) Model for Improvement (MFI) that we use to steer you through the improvement process in practice.

How to get the best out of the book

Reading this chapter first and those following in sequence will ensure you gain the most from this resource, particularly if you are new to quality improvement. Developing a good understanding of the fundamentals outlined in this chapter will provide the foundation you need to develop the integrated, holistic approach to quality improvement that is necessary for success, and a deeper understanding of complex concepts, which will make application of the material in the following chapters easier. Each chapter links to others in the book to enable deeper understanding of key issues as subsequent material and activities build on previous ones. Directions are provided in the text to enable you to track this throughout; for example, how and at which points in the improvement process evaluation needs to be considered and what practical strategies may be employed at each stage.

What is the book about?

The book focuses on leading the quality improvement process from beginning, i.e. identifying a target issue, to end, i.e. sustaining a successful change in practice. It draws on relevant theory and the application of a selection of quality improvement tools and techniques in a healthcare context to enable you to successfully navigate the improvement process. Figure F1 provides the conceptual model of quality improvement we developed and used to guide the structure of the book. This model illustrates the range of theoretical and practical disciplines that successful improvement involves and how these need to be integrated for success; it is derived from theory and our collective experience of facilitating continuous improvement over many years. As is true of any model or visual depiction however, this figure merely provides an overview of the main components. Dotted lines are used to emphasise the interrelated nature and need to integrate the different elements of the model if successful improvement is to be achieved; but this is a simplified depiction and as with most models, is not designed as a stand-alone entity to be used without a deeper understanding of its component parts and how they relate to each other.

The model (Figure F1) builds on the Discipline of Improvement (Penny, 2003), which sits at its core and comprises four interconnected elements. Two of these primarily concern people (i.e. involving service users, carers and staff and personal and organisational development) and two processes (i.e. process and systems thinking and initiating, sustaining and spreading). The Discipline of Improvement (Penny, 2003) provides the broad framework, principles or components for the application or implementation of Improvement Science.

Improvement Science, which may be defined as:

> *exploring how to undertake quality improvement well. It inhabits the sphere between research and quality improvement by applying research methods to help understand what impacts on quality improvement.*

(The Health Foundation, 2011, p3)

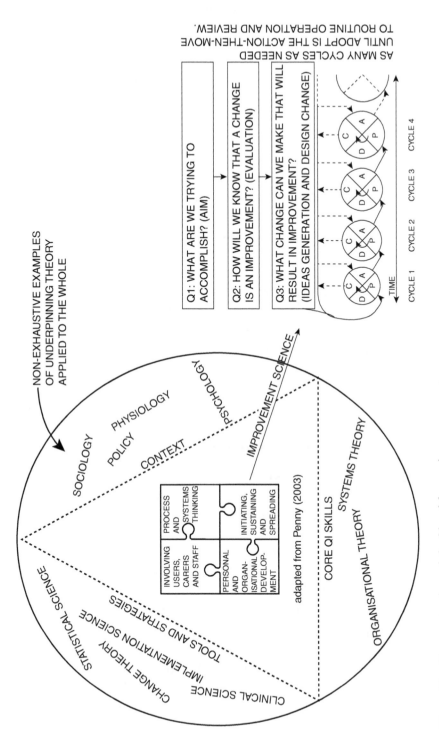

AS MANY CYCLES AS NEEDED
UNTIL ADOPT IS THE ACTION-THEN-MOVE
TO ROUTINE OPERATION AND REVIEW.

Q1: WHAT ARE WE TRYING TO
ACCOMPLISH? (AIM)

Q2: HOW WILL WE KNOW THAT A CHANGE
IS AN IMPROVEMENT? (EVALUATION)

Q3: WHAT CHANGE CAN WE MAKE THAT WILL
RESULT IN IMPROVEMENT?
(IDEAS GENERATION AND DESIGN CHANGE)

TIME

CYCLE 1   CYCLE 2   CYCLE 3   CYCLE 4

NON-EXHAUSTIVE EXAMPLES
OF UNDERPINNING THEORY
APPLIED TO THE WHOLE

PSYCHOLOGY

PHYSIOLOGY

SOCIOLOGY

POLICY

CONTEXT

IMPROVEMENT SCIENCE

PROCESS AND SYSTEMS THINKING

INVOLVING USERS, CARERS AND STAFF

INITIATING, SUSTAINING AND SPREADING

PERSONAL AND ORGAN-ISATIONAL DEVELOP-MENT

adapted from Penny (2003)

CORE QI SKILLS

SYSTEMS THEORY

ORGANISATIONAL THEORY

CLINICAL SCIENCE

IMPLEMENTATION SCIENCE

TOOLS AND STRATEGIES

CHANGE THEORY

STATISTICAL SCIENCE

Figure F1   Conceptual model of healthcare improvement

The Model for Improvement (MFI) (Langley et al, 2009) and the systematic, data driven use of this model to address quality issues or spread best practice has become synonymous with Improvement Science. This has been driven by the Institute for Healthcare improvement's approach to Improvement Science, which they define as:

> *an applied science that emphasises innovation, rapid cycle testing in the field and spread ... to generate learning about what changes, in what contexts produce improvements. It is characterized by the combination of expert subject knowledge with improvement methods and tools. It is multidisciplinary, drawing on clinical science, systems theory, psychology, statistics and other fields.*

(IHI, 2022)

Improvement methods have developed over the years and many of these have been used successfully in the healthcare sector. Each method illustrates the process to follow when facilitating and embedding change to address quality issues or spread best practice. Some are relatively simple and others more complex, but there is no evidence that one is necessarily better than the other (Alderwick et al, 2017). We therefore focus on and use The Model for Improvement (MFI) (Langley et al 2009) as our basis for this book, to guide you through the improvement process in practice. It was designed to support small-scale, emergent, and sustainable change using rapid-cycle testing, learning, and re-testing in the field to enable proximal knowledge generation by and for local health populations and issues (Clarke and Wilcockson, 2002). It is therefore particularly relevant for guiding practitioner led improvement and is commonly used across international and UK healthcare settings to promote sustainable change (see http://www.ihi.org/resources/Pages/HowtoImprove).

The Model for Improvement (MFI) (Langley et al 2009)

The MFI is a structured two-part framework.

Part 1 of the model has three questions:

1. what are we trying to accomplish?
2. how will we know that change represents an improvement?
3. what changes can we make that will lead to improvement?

Responding to the questions forming Part 1 of the MFI lays the foundations for Part 2. It requires developing an improvement aim (question 1), identifying evaluation criteria and measures (question 2) and finally deciding what improvement intervention or change to make (question 3).

Part 2 of the model, the Plan Do Study Act (PDSA) cycle is the implementation stage. Here the changes designed to achieve improvement are planned, implemented and tested against the measures identified in Part 1. The cycle is repeated as the changes are tweaked based on the results of the previous cycle. Unlike research studies, which often measure the impact of interventions using larger sample sizes over a long period of time before confirming the significance of results, Improvement Science uses rapid and initially small-scale testing. This means that learning from the study (evaluation) phase of each cycle is applied to practice in a timely way as refinements are made. The first PDSA cycle, which could involve just one person receiving care, is reviewed and revised based on the data collected, then repeated multiple times. Revisions may include, for example, increasing the number of people involved, testing in different environments, or adjusting an intervention until all stakeholders are satisfied that no further refinements are necessary. This may be because the project aims are met or testing of the changes demonstrates they do not lead to improvement. An example of this in practice is provided in Chapter 5.

One of the main advantages of using the MFI is that evaluation data is generated as you go along and can then be used to guide the next step. This reduces risk and potential waste of resources on good change ideas that for all sorts of reasons will just not work or need adjustments to be successful. Used appropriately the MFI offers a rigorous, experimental approach to improvement, addressing complex improvement problems and responding to the unforeseen impact of change (Reed and Card, 2016). Application of the model involves 'piloting' or testing new ideas rather than wholesale implementation. This **iterative**, cyclical testing and evaluative approach is more likely to achieve **buy-in** or support from colleagues who might otherwise be suspicious or unsupportive of change.

Despite being widely and successfully used in healthcare, the simplicity of the MFI, though highly attractive, belies the complexity involved. This can hinder effective application in practice, particularly by those new to quality improvement. We therefore devised an adapted, more explanatory version (Figure F2) to illustrate in more detail its practical application in practice without changing its fundamental structure or approach; this is used throughout the book as we have found this approach helps others' understanding, particularly when new to improvement.

Our explanatory depiction of the MFI includes four modifications:

- multiple PDSA cycles are depicted to make the iterative testing process more visible. The best way to iterate the cycles to expand the testing/learning in context varies from one improvement to another and is determined by the data/learning from the previous cycle. This introduces a degree of uncertainty as it may not be possible at the start to have more than just a general idea or outline plan of how subsequent cycles will need to evolve. Living with, while managing uncertainty is part of improvement, though Chapter 5 provides an illustrative example of how this might be achieved.
- visual indicators to prompt consideration of the learning from each PDSA within the context of the original purpose, aim and evaluation criteria for the proposed improvement have been added to make this process more visible;
- the 'Study' part of PDSA is replaced with 'Check', which is a later development of the original, though these two terms are often used interchangeably (Taylor et al, 2014). The aim is to more clearly emphasise that the focus of this stage is

on evaluation, i.e. checking the data/results from that cycle against the original purpose, aim, evaluation criteria;

- the importance of considering three possible actions at the 'Act' stage, i.e. abandon, adapt, adopt, is emphasised, with the chosen action being determined by the results of the 'Check' or evaluation element of the current cycle.

You may find it odd that the MFI requires you to consider evaluation (Q2 in Part 1) before identifying what change you intend to make i.e. your aim (Q3 in Part 1). This makes more sense however, if you remember that issues concerning evaluation determining if the change is an improvement or not need to inform the aim.

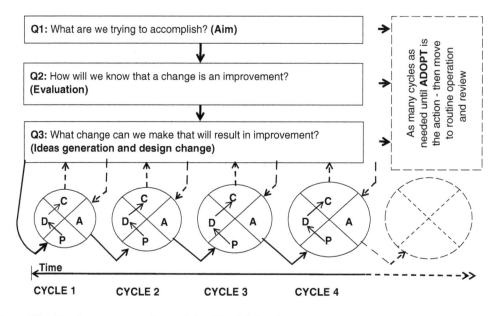

Figure F2   Explanatory version of the Model for Improvement

As with other improvement methods, a variety of tools and techniques are used within each stage of the MFI. These are designed to collect information that will support each stage of the improvement process. For example, at the initial stage of the improvement process the problem being addressed needs to be clearly understood. Tools to support the examination of cause and effect and inter-connected relationships, e.g. Five Whys, Ishikawa (Fishbone diagram) and Process or Value Stream Mapping are often used to help with this; others include Lewin's Force Field Analysis, which looks at drivers for and against change (see the further reading section at the end of this chapter for more information on a wide range of improvement tools).

Some tools are used in different ways at different project stages. For example, when we meet Harry in Chapter 1 you will see stakeholder identification used during the initial stages to discover the key stakeholders involved with his improvement idea (see Chapters 1, 2 and 5). As the improvement process progresses, stakeholder analysis is used to explore the interests and priorities of those involved or affected by the proposed improvement or changes being introduced (see Chapters 2, 3 and 5). This analysis informs the development of a stakeholder management and communication plan that promotes effective continued engagement and communication about the improvement, with everyone involved (see Chapters 3, 5 and 6). It is very important that the needs of different stakeholders continue to be met as the project moves forward and the plan facilitates this.

Tools and strategies for improvement therefore form one side of the 'triangle' surrounding the core of the conceptual model (Figure F1) used to guide the structure of the book overall as these are applied throughout the improvement process. The other sides of the 'triangle' comprise 'leadership' and 'context' because the application of these concepts also affects the whole of the improvement process. For example, the effectiveness of the application of a particular improvement tool may be just as dependent on the leadership approach adopted when using it as the suitability or quality of the tool itself. This can mean the difference between success and failure; therefore, it is addressed in more depth in Chapters 2 and 6. Similarly, any improvement idea or activity takes places within a particular context; as you will see in Chapter 2, healthcare is a complex adaptive system involving the interaction of innumerable factors. These may include, for example, professional, societal and clinical or organisational issues at individual, local, national or international level that each have a bearing on the improvement itself and must all be considered as part of any change proposition.

The final, outer component of the conceptual model in Figure F1 comprises the 'soup' of different disciplines and theories in which any improvement activity needs to be immersed for success. The theories identified are key examples rather than an exhaustive list and will be addressed in more detail in specific chapters. For example, see Chapter 2 for an explanation of systems theory or Chapter 3 for a detailed discussion of change theory. Other topics such as clinical science and psychology are infused throughout the book.

Differentiating quality improvement from audit and research

These three activities all play a role in improving the quality of care and often involve using similar processes, systems and methods but have quite different purposes and regulatory requirements, so being able to differentiate between them is crucial. Quality improvement is a data-guided activity that often involves humans and sometimes uses methods that are also used in health research and audit; therefore, it is wholly appropriate and not surprising that its relationship to ethical and governance standards for the protection of human research subjects arises. The UK Health Research Authority decision tool and associated guidance is easily accessible and should be used at the outset to help you determine the status of your quality improvement proposal and the type of ethical and governance approvals required. You should also take advice from your lecturer and the relevant experts in your employing organisation. Different organisations use different labels but you will find these experts in departments such as Research and

Development, Research and Innovation, Clinical Audit and your project supervisor (lecturer) should also be able to signpost you to the right people for advice.

We all have an important role in ensuring any improvement activity is conducted in a safe and ethical manner (Dixon, 2021) while also accounting for other relevant factors. For example, all healthcare professionals also have an obligation to improve the quality and safety of care; therefore while aiming to uphold the ethical principles of informed consent and voluntary participation as you would for research, the traditional research approach to consent may not be wholly appropriate for staff participating in some quality improvements (Baily et al, 2006). This highlights the inherent tension and pragmatic balance that must be struck between the rights and responsibilities of health staff and is just one example of why the theory and practice of ethical and governance oversight of quality improvement remains a contested issue (Cribb et al, 2020). See Figure F3, which identifies the steps you can take to apply good practice.

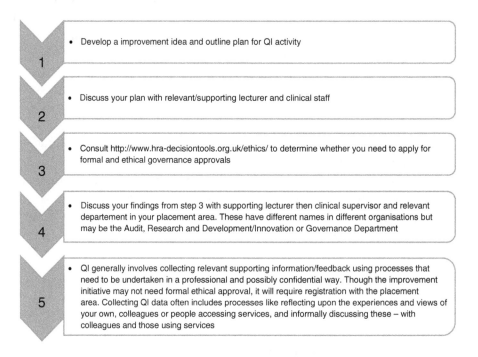

Figure F3   Steps to take when implementing QI activity in practice

Clinical audit may be defined as a 'systematic review of care against explicit criteria and as such is a quality improvement process' (Dixon, 2021, p5). As illustrated in Chapter 4, it is often used when analysing a practice issue to determine whether change is required and can help to clarify which change option is most appropriate while also providing a pre-change baseline measure to inform subsequent evaluation. You may also have come across evaluation projects that use activities and methods commonly associated with research, but because they are evaluating a service against specific service aims or standards they are classified as service evaluation rather than research. Working out the status of an improvement project can be complex but, regardless, you will need to secure approvals as appropriate for an improvement project. Commonly, university research ethics and governance systems and processes are used to support scrutiny of improvement projects, though this often requires some adaptation. As a student, you will need to have your project approved by the university, who will normally require evidence of project registration and approval in principle from the research and development department of the organisation in which the project is taking place, along with the HRA decision tool outcome.

The way a project is framed and the terminology used is important to enable you to maintain the appropriate improvement focus. For example, the term project proposal is commonly used for an improvement project outline or plan, whereas the equivalent for a research study or project is termed a protocol; you are also likely to be gathering staff feedback on the project process and outcomes as part of the 'Check' stage of the Plan Do Check Act (PDCA) and the evaluation of your improvement, rather than conducting staff interviews or focus groups, and therefore require different ethical or governance approval. However, in practice, terms are often used interchangeably, which can be confusing.

Chapter summary

This chapter has provided the information needed to help you develop a good understanding of the fundamental concepts of quality improvement and how to get the best out of this book. You should now be ready to move on to consider in more detail what quality improvement is and why it is important for you and nursing more generally.

Glossary

Iterative: doing something repeatedly, usually using minor changes each time to improve the outcome
Buy-in: the extent to which others are supportive of change

Further reading

Batalden, P and Davidoff, F (2006) Introduction to quality improvement: What is 'quality improvement' and how can it transform healthcare? *BMJ Quality & Safety*, http://dx.doi.org/10.1136/qshc.2006.022046

Useful websites

http://www.hra-decisiontools.org.uk/ethics/ UK Health Research Authority (n.d.) Do I Need NHS REC Review?

http://www.ihi.org/resources/Pages/HowtoImproveScienceofImprovementEstablishingMeasures.aspx Institute for Healthcare Improvement (n.d.) *Science of Improvement: Improving Measures* – useful information on differentiating measures for QI from those for research.

https://bit.ly/3Nkp1l9 NHS England – further information on quality, service improvement and redesign.

https://bit.ly/3Ogvvmp Quality Improvement Zone – further information on a wide range of QI tools.

https://www.youtube.com/watch?app=desktop&v=NyHxRJLM-0s An overview of quality improvement, with Dr Mareeni Raymond.

Part 1

Establishing the context: Introducing Harry

Catherine Delves-Yates and Gillian Janes

This first part of the textbook will enable you to understand what quality improvement is, and why it is so important in nursing. We will be considering the role of quality improvement in person-centred care, understanding the terminology used and, most importantly, starting to recognise how quality improvement can become a feature of our everyday practice.

At the start of each chapter, you will hear from registered nurses and nursing students, who are very likely to be sharing the challenges and asking the questions you are as you work upon developing your quality improvement skills. Before you start to read the chapters in this part, however, we would like to introduce you to Harry Anand, who is going to share his thoughts about an idea where current practice could be improved. As we progress through this part of the book we will refer back to Harry and identify how he could develop his idea further.

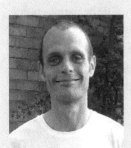

Hi! My name is Harry Anand. I am 19 and a first-year nursing student, currently in the second week of my first placement experience. I have always wanted to be a nurse. I am very interested in learning how to support patients with long-term conditions, and how it is possible for them to continue with their daily life despite their illness.

While I was doing my A levels I did some work experience in a GP surgery – sadly I didn't get to do very much with the patients, I mainly helped with booking appointments and learning how to keep the electronic record for each patient up to date. It was very interesting though and made me realise how much information is collected about patients.

In my current placement I am fully involved in caring for patients, which is something I am really excited about. There is so much to learn though, and even though we did lots of skills practice before starting placement, I am feeling totally overwhelmed by everything. On my

(Continued)

(Continued)

first day I could easily have just hidden in the sluice! I am enjoying most of it though, even though it is very nerve wracking. I am worried that something will happen and I won't know what to do.

I need lots of support from my supervisor, but I am slowly starting to understand the daily routine. I have been getting lots of practice of taking patients' observations and recording them on the correct chart. Doing this is really helpful – taking a patient's blood pressure manually is something I need lots of practise with, as I am finding it difficult because I don't always manage to hear them!

Unlike the GP surgery where I did work experience, patient observations on the ward are not recorded electronically, they are all written on paper. I was really surprised to find this, so I did some investigation to see whether this is the case in lots of wards. This also allowed me to put into action what we have learnt so far in school about searching for literature!! According to a Freedom of Information request reported by Health Europa (2019), in 2019 only 1 in 10 NHS Trusts were fully digitised, plus an article in the *British Medical Journal* (Iacobucci, 2020) said that the plans to fully digitise the NHS over the next ten years are unlikely to be achieved without further investment. So, it looks as if it might still be a few more years until all patient observations are recorded electronically, rather than on pieces of paper and kept in folders at the patients' bedside.

When I am recording the observations, one thing I keep thinking about is the amount of other information there is in the folder at each patients' bedside. There is so much of it. I am not sure all of it needs to be there. Some of the folders are absolutely crammed full, and the information goes back over quite a few weeks. Also, there doesn't seem to be any specific order in the way information is filed in the folder, each one seems to be organised differently. This makes it difficult for me to find the correct chart to record the patient observations on. I am a bit worried about this, because what would happen if we needed to find this information quickly? One of the patients yesterday became unexpectedly unwell, and the doctor wanted to know what their observations were. It was lucky that I had just finished recording the observations, so I knew where to find the chart. If I hadn't just written on it, I wouldn't have been able to find it so quickly.

Thinking back to my experience in the GP surgery, it was so easy to find what was needed in the electronic patient records. I think it would be possible to do something similar with the paper records though – they can be kept in a more organised way. We could ensure that every folder had the same order of information, with the different sections clearly identified by dividers. I think that if we had a standard way of organising the patient bedside files, it would make things very much easier.

Now, I am unsure what I should do about this idea. It probably isn't important so I should concentrate upon learning about how to care for patients rather than worrying about folders! In School, however, we were told to always talk to our supervisor if we were concerned about anything. I am a bit concerned about how much of a muddle the folders at the patient bedsides are, but my supervisor is always so busy, and she might think I was wasting her time by talking to her about it. Surely the staff will have thought about this before – it is such a small thing. I am so new to caring for patients, with much to learn. I think it is likely that I am not focusing upon the right thing. I should be practising my skills rather than worrying about things like patient bedside folders.

However, making changes to how we organise them and reducing how much 'stuff' there is in each one would make recording observations quicker and make it easier to find things in an emergency. So maybe I should say something ...?

Chapter 1

What is quality improvement and why is it important?

Gillian Janes and Catherine Delves-Yates

Chapter aims

After reading this chapter you should be able to:

- identify **key drivers** for quality improvement in healthcare;
- use **contemporary** quality improvement terminology appropriately;
- understand the role of stakeholders and the importance of engaging them from the start;
- reflect on the nurse's role in and nursing's contribution to quality improvement;
- apply the principles of **innovation** within your practice as a nursing student.

I just don't understand why the last year of my nursing programme seems to focus so much upon quality improvement. Is it really relevant to my role as a nursing student and then as a newly qualified nurse – surely this information is for managers?

(Jyothi, 3rd year nursing student)

I am reading about quality improvement – but there are so many new terms to understand! How can I get to grips with them?

(Dave, registered nurse)

Introduction

Quality improvement is a topic that is frequently discussed in relation to many aspects of healthcare. As Jyothi tells us at the start of the chapter, it is also a subject that forms part of the learning in both pre-registration and post-registration nursing programmes. In this chapter we are going to consider why this is the case.

At the moment you may share Jyothi's difficulty in appreciating how quality improvement can be seen as an integral aspect of the knowledge needed to care for people effectively. It could also be that, like Dave, who we also heard from at the start of the chapter, you are struggling to understand the language of quality improvement. To help you build a strong foundation for your quality improvement knowledge, in this chapter we are going to outline the fundamental role quality improvement has in enabling you to deliver the best care possible to service users. Firstly, we will discuss what quality improvement is, and the reasons why it is important in healthcare. We will then consider how it is possible to understand the many new words you will encounter when reading about quality improvements. The importance of not working in isolation when undertaking quality improvement will be highlighted, and finally we will identify how you can adopt an innovative approach to the care you deliver.

Quality improvement in context: the strategic agenda

Quality improvement in healthcare is not new, having been propelled in the United Kingdom by various national health and social care policies and initiatives over the last 20–30 years. This is in response to examples of serious clinical performance issues like with children's heart surgery at the Bristol Royal Infirmary; individual criminal cases and lack of oversight such as that of General Practitioner Harold Shipman; and the public inquiries that followed them. The latter example led to changes to the revalidation of doctors and health professions more widely, signifying a move from self to professional regulation with a focus on safety. Subsequent failings by health organisations and systems, for example in acute services (Francis, 2013), learning disability (Heslop et al, 2013) and maternity services (Ockenden 2022) have continued, however. Meanwhile, national health and social care policies have changed over this time, moving from an emphasis on improving the person centredness of care and developing service user-led services, to quality assurance, to improving service user safety. These changes continue today; for example, the Five Year Forward View (NHS England 2014) outlined three main areas in which the NHS needed to meet the changing needs of the population, one of which was improving the quality of care. This led to the development of sustainability and transformation plans across England to provide more detail on what local changes were needed in all parts of the NHS (Alderwick and Ham, 2017) to make this vision a reality (Ham et al, 2017).

What drives these policies is the need to respond to the societal and scientific changes that continue to result in an increasing demand for more complex and flexible care as well as increased organisational accountability and transparency. This is against the backdrop of an ageing population and increasing public expectations fuelled by advances in science and technology, despite the limited financial resources and serious workforce supply and skills gap facing the healthcare sector (MacDonald, 2020).

But why and how should high level government policy concern nurses? The relevance of quality improvement as a practical concept for busy nurses was highlighted almost two decades ago by the NHS Institute for Innovation and Improvement:

> *Every single person is enabled, encouraged and capable to work with others to improve their part of the service.*

> (Penny, 2003)

And it remains true today. This assertion, that all staff have a role to play in ensuring that healthcare services continue to improve, was reiterated more recently by The Health Foundation (THF) in *Quality Improvement Made Simple* (2021) and steps have been taken to make this a requirement for all healthcare staff. For example, quality improvement is a core dimension of the NHS Knowledge and Skills Framework (DH, 2004) and is an integral part of the nursing role that explicitly features in many job descriptions. This includes, for example, those for newly qualified practitioners, as employers seek staff who can not only do the job but can also contribute to improving that job for the benefit of service users, colleagues and the wider organisation. It should therefore come as no surprise to you that improvement is the focus of Platform 6 'Improving the safety and quality of care' in the NMC Standards of Proficiency for Registered Nurses (NMC, 2018a).

Hindering progress in improving the quality of NHS services, however, is the lack of a single, coherent national strategy for how to implement improvement (Ham et al, 2016). Thus, while improving the quality of healthcare remains a priority, the implementation of this is feeble (Molloy et al, 2016) and patchy. While healthcare system-wide improvement is required but not often achieved, there are many examples across the NHS of successful, relatively small-scale quality improvement initiatives as illustrated by the Case study later in this chapter. These are often designed and implemented by teams working at the front line and have led to significant benefits for service users and staff, while also delivering better value (Alderwick et al, 2017).

It is therefore important that all nurses are engaged and equipped to undertake small-scale improvements as part of their normal everyday practice. The national improvement framework (NHS Improvement, 2016) goes some way to enabling this by outlining key steps and resources for supporting improvement capability building and leadership development in NHS services. This framework is designed to support the development of knowledge of improvement methods and how to use them at all levels of the NHS. It also emphasises the importance of developing leadership skills alongside improvement knowledge to achieve this. In our experience, the simultaneous development of these two skills is crucial for successful improvement. This explains why you will see that as you progress through these chapters, the key leadership skills associated with each part of the improvement process are also addressed and you are strongly advised to refer to the sister title in the TNP series (Ellis, 2019) to further develop your leadership knowledge. Thus, it is recognised that frontline staff engaged in improvement need to develop the skills required to identify quality problems, carry out tests of change, measure their impact and act on the results (Alderwick et al, 2017). Before going on to explore these skills in more detail, however, we must first define what is meant by quality improvement.

Key definitions and terminology explained

Quality improvement focuses on

making healthcare safe, effective, service user-centred, timely, efficient and equitable.

(THF, 2021, p7)

and involves

the systematic use of tools and methods to continuously improve quality of care and outcomes for patients.

(Alderwick et al, 2017, p1)

But what is quality and how is this defined in terms of healthcare? The hugely influential framework proposed by the Institute of Medicine (IOM) Report (2001) identifies six domains of healthcare system quality, which are outlined in Figure 1.1. The acronym TEPEES (Timely, Effective, Person-centred, Efficient, Equitable, Safe) (The Health Foundation, 2021) may help you memorise them.

Safe	• Avoiding harm to patients from care that is intended to help them.
Effective	• Providing services based in scientific knowledge to all who could benefit and refraining from providing services to those not likely to benefit (avoiding overuse and underuse respectively).
Patient-centred	• Providing care that is respectful and responsive to individual patient preferences, needs and values, and ensuring that patient values guide all clinical decisions.
Timely	• Reducing waits and sometimes harmful delays for both those who recieve and those who give care.
Efficient	• Avoiding waste, including waste of equipment, supplies, ideas and energy.
Equitable	• Providing care that does not vary in quality because of personal characteristics such as gender, ethnicity, geographic location and socioeconomic status.

Figure 1.1   The six domains of healthcare system quality (IOM, 2001)

Do these domains seem familiar to you? They are reflected in the aims of the NHS Constitution (DH, 2009), which include ensuring high quality, free NHS services, value for money for the taxpayer and the values that underpin this, such as a commitment to the quality of care. The IOM (2001) quality domains are also explicitly echoed in the NMC Code (NMC 2018b), particularly the standards, which require all nurses to prioritise people, practice effectively and promote safety.

The NMC Code (2018b) clearly outlines how we must prioritise people, practice effectively and promote safety. Read about Daniel's improvement – Improving person-centred care in General Practice in the case study below – to see how this can be done.

Case study   Improving person-centred care in General Practice

Daniel was on placement in a General Practice. It was very different to working in the hospital but he was enjoying the experience. The normally friendly atmosphere was spoiled one day when the community nurse was complaining about unnecessary multiple visits for Laurie, who had complex needs. Daniel discovered that community nurse visits had been requested on consecutive days for different blood tests when the samples could all have been taken at the same time. This would not only have reduced the community nurse workload but would have been much better for Laurie as he would only have needed one venepuncture; this was especially important as he had an aversion to needles and became very upset. Daniel had noticed that the practice team used a whiteboard to share information and community nurse visit requests, which helped the team co-ordinate visits. He was surprised, however, to find that this system was not normally used to request visits for blood tests. Daniel asked why the whiteboard wasn't used for this type of visit request – after all, the board was in a staff area and only visible to practice staff so there would be no confidentiality issue. His colleague wasn't sure, so together they raised it at the next staff meeting and discovered that the whiteboard had been introduced for a different reason and using it to co-ordinate venepuncture visit requests had never been suggested. Given the unnecessary distress caused to Laurie and the potential for saving community nurse time, it was agreed to trial collating visit requests for blood samples on the whiteboard to ensure all relevant samples could be taken at one visit, and to review how this new system was working at the weekly practice meetings.

As Daniel's case study illustrates, nursing and healthcare are **human-centric,** team-based endeavours and as such, rely on effective communication. The shared professional language of quality improvement we use is crucial for enabling the common understanding necessary for the complex interpersonal communication that underpins the delivery of high quality care. You will already be increasing your familiarity with much of the medical and technical terminology associated with nursing practice. This will encompass human anatomy, e.g. xiphisternum, clinical equipment, e.g. sphygmomanometer and clinical processes, e.g. percutaneous endoscopic gastronomy. In quality improvement it is common, however, for different terms to be used when referring to the same thing, even by colleagues in the same organisation: professional background further complicates this. In addition, you may come across specific improvement methods or approaches, e.g. Time to Care, Kaizen or service transformation without recognising these as such. As Figure 1.2 shows, one of the challenges of quality improvement is that it can seem like a whole new language at first; accessing and becoming familiar with the shared professional language of quality improvement can be a real challenge.

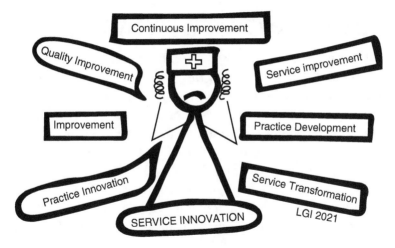

Figure 1.2   The same thing?

Often the terms highlighted in Figure 1.2 are used interchangeably, and this is not an exhaustive list. While there may be nuanced differences in meaning, all these terms broadly refer to a process of improvement outlined earlier. In the interests of clarity therefore, we will use 'improvement' as a general term representing the myriad of associated names. Referring to the glossary at the end of each chapter where necessary as you read will also help to develop your understanding of the meaning of improvement terminology. You will also find it useful to collate and refer to your own improvement vocabulary resource as you progress; Activity 1.1 guides you through this process.

Activity 1.1   Building knowledge

Think about the improvement related terms you have come across in your placement(s), or the organisation(s) you have worked in, your reading or other sources.

Start recording these using your chosen method, by:

- jotting them down in a notebook;
- keeping a list on your laptop or phone;
- keeping an 'Improvement' vocabulary book;
- making an audio memo.

You will find it most helpful to record the term itself, what you understand the term to mean and an example of where/when you have seen it used. Discuss anything you are unclear about with your practice supervisor, university lecturer or someone with an interest or role in improvement. This might be a colleague who has led an improvement project in your placement area, a final year student completing an improvement project or a member of your organisation's improvement/transformation team. Keep adding new terms to your 'improvement vocabulary resource' as you meet them and use it to remind yourself what the terms mean. This will deepen your understanding throughout your career as you develop your improvement expertise.

As this activity is based on your own work, there is no outline answer at the end of the chapter.

Who does improvement involve?

We have considered what drives improvement, what the term means, its importance as a core nursing skill and the value it adds. But who does this added value benefit? The answer may depend upon the improvement in question and its context but, in general, there will be many more individuals and groups for whom a single improvement adds value than you might imagine! It is natural that those likely to experience immediate or direct benefit, e.g. service users and their families, staff or the local clinical area might first come to mind or be easiest to identify. It is also likely, however, that many others who might not be obvious could also benefit indirectly. For example, improving the way care is delivered for one service user has the potential to influence the care of others in the same or other wards or settings and eventually many others by influencing national policy change. Such changes also add value to the organisation, for example by enhancing effectiveness or organisational reputation in terms of service user satisfaction ratings or staff wellbeing. Eventually, such developments can add value at a higher level, impacting, for example, wider society in terms of general population health or public confidence.

You may already have come across the term stakeholders. Taken literally this simply means anyone who has a stake in a particular issue or the outcome. The first consideration concerns who the stakeholders are for any given improvement, before going on to analyse how they might most meaningfully be engaged in the improvement process. This second step is often termed stakeholder analysis and is important as it guides how we interact and communicate with these individuals and groups to achieve the most appropriate and sustainable outcome. It is well recognised that for the best chance of success, the widest possible range of people and groups that are either affected by the improvement idea being explored or would be required to behave differently for a change to be successful are at least consulted and at best involved from the very start.

Activity 1.2   Reflection

Would you agree with the statement:

It is well recognised that for the best chance of success, the widest possible range of people and groups that are either affected by the improvement idea being explored or would be required to behave differently for a change to be successful are at least consulted and at best involved from the very start.

- If so, why is this?
- If not, what are your reasons for this?

Take a few minutes to reflect upon your view relating to these questions and what has influenced this, then talk to your peers or practice supervisor about what they think.

As this activity is based on your own reflection, there is no outline answer at the end of the chapter.

It is important to take a systematic approach and be as comprehensive as possible when identifying stakeholders; we may otherwise miss a specific perspective or some crucial information that could be the key to arriving at the best solution or smoothing the change process.

Activity 1.3   Measuring

Look back to the start of Part 1 and Harry's reflection on the problem he identified with the service users' bedside records format. Harry did mention it to his practice supervisor, who was very supportive and suggested they could explore what could be done to improve matters.

To start the stakeholder analysis process, take a sheet of paper and write Harry's idea in the centre. Then jot down around this all the individuals or groups that Harry and his practice supervisor would need to consider if they are to take this matter forward. Perhaps start with the immediate team but don't forget to think more widely than this in terms of who might need to be involved in any change and/or who else might be interested in what they are doing. Then, think about the different levels of involvement and commitment required from each of these stakeholders and depict this on your paper – you can do this in any way you choose, for example, using thicker/thinner/dotted lines to connect each stakeholder to Harry's idea at the centre.

Once you've done this compare your analysis with the activity answer at the end of the chapter to see if we agree.

Each improvement idea and the environment it occurs in will be slightly different, but thinking in this way will help you to develop the habit of considering the potential stakeholders in any given situation, which will definitely increase your chances of improvement success. Successful stakeholder engagement has been identified as a core improvement skill (Lucas and Nacer, 2015) and, as such, can make all the difference to the success of your improvement efforts. It is closely related to your leadership skills and ability to work effectively with others, which we will consider further when we return to the topic of stakeholders in forthcoming chapters.

'Being innovative'

'Innovation' and 'being innovative' are words that we are used to hearing frequently in respect of many areas of our lives. If you question what the precise meaning of these frequently used terms is, however, it is very easy to become confused. Innovation is a word often used in connection with not only healthcare, but education, technology, business and much more. Often innovation is associated with scientific breakthroughs and ground-breaking research, but innovation encompasses more than just large-scale, life changing discovery.

The simplest way to think about innovation is as something new and original; the word 'innovative' originates from the Latin word 'novus', which means new. This provides a good starting point for consideration of the term – an innovation is something new, which changes the way we do things; although, there is yet further potential confusion, because if we define innovation in this way, how does it differ from an invention? There is a sound way to differentiate between the two, highlighting a really important aspect of innovation, or being innovative. To truly be described as an innovation, what we are referring to needs to 'create value'. So, not only is there a difference between innovation and invention, but we can complete our simple definition by concluding that innovation is:

> *something new, which changes the way we do things in a way that is valuable.*

While our simple definition is getting close to fully explaining the term, it is not yet perfect. As outlined in Figure 1.3, there are still a few questions to consider.

- Does an innovation have to be new to the entire world, or just those who are benefitting from it?

- Who needs to value an innovation? The entire world, or just those who are experiencing it?

- What do we mean by value – is this purely monetary, or, in respect of healthcare especially, can value be improving people's experience of healthcare?

Figure 1.3   Questions to consider …

Activity 1.4   Reflection

Thinking about Figure 1.3 Questions to consider … How would you fully define innovation? Make a note of your personal definition, then check the activity answers at the end of the chapter and ask your peers or practice supervisor, to see whether their thoughts are similar.

There are outline answers to this activity at the end of the chapter.

While finding a truly objective way to decide whether something is an innovation can cause a great deal of head scratching, there is a good source of guidance focusing upon healthcare innovation. The World Health Organisation (WHO) (2021a) defines innovation in healthcare as new or improved health policies, systems, products, technologies, services and delivery methods that improve health and wellbeing. So, while healthcare innovations come in many different forms, they all share the end result (or outcome) of improving health. WHO (2021a) also outlines that healthcare innovation can be in response to unmet public health needs, which involve creating new ways of thinking and working to address the care required by vulnerable populations. So, innovations can be both improvements to current healthcare and/or new ways of delivering care, specifically to improve access to care for those whom current services do not reach. If we think back to the questions relating to creating value, WHO (2021a) provides us with an answer, by stating value is added by improving the efficiency, effectiveness, quality, sustainability, safety and/or affordability of healthcare. This clearly reflects the six domains of healthcare system quality identified by The Institute of Medicine Report (2001) presented in Figure 1.1; therefore, the WHO (2021a) and The Institute of Medicine Report (2001) both identify that:

1. innovation can happen in all areas of healthcare;
2. we can all be innovative in our practice by reviewing our actions and making changes that improve the outcome.

As we mentioned, innovation is often thought of as being life changing for the entire population. If we consider the introduction of the wheel, it most certainly changed travel across the globe, adding both monetary and social value to people's lives. For most of us, however, trying to introduce innovation upon a worldwide scale is not something we can achieve. Fortunately, it is also the case that innovation can occur upon a small scale. Just a slight change that improves a minor aspect of the care we deliver to service users on a ward, for example, not only qualifies as innovation, but is important.

Thinking further about 'being innovative' in our everyday practice, Thomas Edison (1847–1931) the American inventor, has some advice – 'There's a way to do it better. Find it.' Have you thought that there could be a better way to deliver care to service users? Whenever you think this, make the most of it, write it down and talk to the others involved in the situation. Gaining the perspective of others at an early stage is very helpful as they are likely to have relevant thoughts and experiences.

Working in this way, constantly thinking about how what you are doing could be better, enables you to 'be innovative' in all your activities. While innovation can be ground-breaking and have an impact across the whole globe, it can also occur in small steps in relation to everyday activities. Never underestimate the power of small. If we all constantly generate small innovations, when they are combined, the outcome is improvement upon a grand scale.

Developing an improvement mind-set

The type of thinking outlined in 'Being innovative' could be described as an 'improvement mind-set'. A person's mind-set is their way of thinking and general attitude to things (Collins Dictionary, 2021). Mind-set theory, developed by Carol Dweck, is a way of understanding to what extent an individual perceives the factors associated with a concept as being instinctive and stable ('fixed' mind-set) or variable and potentially influenced ('growth' mind-set) (Wolcott et al, 2020). Investigating an individual's mind-set reveals core beliefs about a concept or topic. Activity 1.5 encourages you to explore your current mind-set regarding improvement.

Activity 1.5   Reflection

Think about what improvement means to you and notice what comes to mind. Do you see it as:

- something that others (usually improvement specialists or the transformation team) do?
- just something else that nurses must focus on when the priority should be developing their core nursing and technical skills?
- a set of tools and frameworks – some of which, e.g. The Model for Improvement or the NHS Change Model, nurses are familiar with, while others, e.g. Lean Methodology or Complex Adaptive Systems, seem like management tools designed to save costs and are written in another language entirely?
- a different discipline that nurses might specialise in later in their career?
- something else ...?

As this activity is based on your own reflection, there is no outline answer at the end of the chapter.

The prompts in Activity 1.5 What does 'improvement' mean to me? Illustrate some of the attitudes and beliefs commonly expressed by nurses and other healthcare staff. As improvement capability has been considered a core skill for all healthcare staff for many years, however, it is important to reflect on how and by what your attitudes and beliefs have been influenced.

The strategic context of improvement outlined earlier in the chapter makes it clear that an improvement mind-set is considered a core aspect of being a good nurse and should be a routine aspect of everyday practice. This view is in line with the NMC Code (2018b), particularly in respect of Prioritising People, Practising Effectively and Promoting Safety. It also reflects the NHS values (DH, 2009), specifically those of 'commitment to quality of care' and 'improving lives' through enhancing people's wellbeing and experiences of the NHS.

Your individual contribution to improvement will vary depending on your stage of professional development and the specific context in which you are working. As a nursing student, the improvement issues you choose to focus on would normally be at an individual service user level initially, but this small (micro) focus may widen to the team or service (meso) level or even an organisational, national or international (macro) perspective as you progress.

Of all healthcare staff, nurses spend arguably the most time in direct interaction with people accessing health services. We also work with a wide range of other multidisciplinary team (MDT) members, so are in a unique position to identify aspects of care delivery that work extremely well or would benefit from improvement. Recognising and cultivating an 'improvement mind-set' is key to maximising the contribution of nursing to improving service delivery and the resulting experiences and health-related outcomes for people.

Nursing students particularly have a unique opportunity to develop and use an improvement mind-set to enable change and spread excellent practice. The temporary nature of practice placements means that nursing students experience each placement area with 'fresh eyes'. This is a key skill for improvers and, coupled with curiosity and a willingness to share with others what you notice, is the essence of an improvement mind-set. Within approximately six months of working in a clinical area, staff become accustomed to the local environment and work culture. This makes it much more difficult to notice aspects of the environment or care delivery that are good or would benefit from improvement. This is one reason why proactive, forward-thinking care teams value and support nursing students working in their areas, but also illustrates how you can use what can be a challenging situation, i.e. regularly joining and leaving different teams, for the benefit of service users, families, healthcare colleagues and your own skills development.

Developing an improvement mind-set starts with becoming alert to 'triggers for improvement'. This is achieved by using your core nursing skills of observation or listening, reflection and empathy to notice how and how effectively individual service users and family needs are being addressed. There are formal ways of identifying 'triggers for improvement', including audits, service user feedback or staff surveys. However, very impactful improvements can arise from just listening to service user or colleague experiences as you go about your normal everyday work. There is plenty of scope for this type of improvement. For example, the '15secs30mins' initiative involves healthcare staff identifying how they could spend a few extra seconds on a task to save someone else 30 minutes or more later and was begun by a clinician who came up with the idea while tidying up at home. This approach and the many examples of its application in practice has had a big impact on reducing staff frustration and increasing joy at work, which we know ultimately results in better service user care. To find out more visit http://15s30m.co.uk/ for examples from real NHS staff. Activity 1.6 will also help you to identify triggers for improvement in your practice.

Activity 1.6   Observation

a.   **Listening to service user/carer stories**

Talk to 2–3 service users or carers in your area about their views of the care/service they have experienced. Listen to their descriptions of their experiences of accessing/receiving care. What do these descriptions tell us about their experience? What positives that they identify should be maintained? What issues or areas of concern did they raise? What

(Continued)

(Continued)

themes emerge from these descriptions? What are the implications of this for practice and possible improvement?

b. Observations of practice and listening to colleagues

Be alert to what you see and hear around you. You might notice certain practices that seem to cause difficulty or frustration for staff – often they will comment on these in passing. You might notice something where another way of working, or of changing something quite simple, could have a useful impact.

Do any themes emerge from these activities in respect of ideas for improvement? Talk to your practice supervisor or university lecturer about how you might develop this.

NB: This is NOT an 'interviewing' or formal observation exercise but IS about taking notice of what you see and hear as you go about your everyday role. The focus is on service user/carer and staff experience of receiving or delivering care.

As this activity is based on your own observation, there is no outline answer at the end of the chapter.

In Activity 1.6 Identifying 'triggers for improvement', the idea of looking for themes within information is considered. Read about Saraya's improvement – Reducing 'Did not attend' (DNAs) in an outpatient clinic in the case study below to see how useful this can be.

Case study Reducing 'Did not attend' (DNAs) in an outpatient clinic

Saraya was on placement in outpatients. She was surprised by what seemed to her to be a large number of DNAs for one particular clinic, so she mentioned what she had noticed to her practice assessor one day when they were discussing how she had settled in. The assessor suggested she investigate further and put her in touch with a colleague who could help her access the attendance numbers for that particular clinic. The pattern she noticed in the figures surprised Saraya. What she discovered when she looked at the number of DNAs for each day of the week was that these were much more numerous on Mondays, Thursdays and Fridays. However, she also noticed that, week after week, the majority of DNAs on Mondays were younger people (20–30 years) and those at the end of the week were mostly older people (65+ years). Saraya shared her discovery with her practice assessor, who suggested they discuss what she had found with the manager and appointments lead. Together they decided to trial scheduling appointments for younger people later on in the week and older people at the start to see if that made any difference. To their surprise the number of DNAs dropped from approximately 30% to 10% and this was still the case a few weeks later.

In a busy clinic running every day, this improvement made a big difference. Appointments were therefore routinely scheduled like this from then on and they continued to monitor the numbers of DNAs, which stayed low. Saraya was asked to share what she had done at one of the Trust's regular 'improvement celebrations' and presented a poster outlining this improvement at the RCN conference, where colleagues facing similar challenges in reducing high DNA rates were keen to talk to her about what she'd done so they could try it.

Astonishment reporting is a tool used by many non-healthcare organisations to benefit from the 'fresh eyes' approach to identify valuable, current practices that should be maintained and support continuous improvement. This approach is now starting to be used by senior healthcare staff with their practice teams, students in evaluation of their nursing programme, to enhance the experience of new lecturers, and Vigier and Bryant (2009) used it to support student reflection upon their learning experience.

Astonishment reporting involves individuals identifying things that astonish them (about the team/organisation or their work) as being excellent or needing development. The format of an 'Astonishment Report' is flexible but should be succinct and specific – usually a bullet point list – which is then reviewed during an exploratory conversation between the new staff member and an established member of the team (ideally not the line manager), to ensure clarity and explore potential actions.

Collation of these reports enables teams/organisations to identify emerging themes and prioritise potential improvement activities. It also provides an opportunity to re-examine and perhaps reaffirm why some processes/procedures are as they are, which can be just as beneficial for the team/organisation as well as the individual completing the report.

Activity 1.7   Measuring

Complete an 'Astonishment Report' based on a previous placement or as part of your contribution to the next one and explore with your practice supervisor or university lecturer how you might share this with the clinical team.

A sample report is provided at the end of the chapter.

Although identifying a potential improvement is important, this is only part of the mind-set needed to spread excellent practice and achieve improvement. You may now be able to see a better future, i.e. have a vision, but action will be required to turn this into reality. To achieve this you will need to draw on your personal qualities and leadership skills; such as being proactive, communicating effectively, working with and influencing others, gathering and evaluating data. These are transferable skills that you are already developing and using in other aspects of your nursing role such as working as part of a multidisciplinary team or educating service users and families. Developing your improvement expertise is therefore integrated with other aspects of your development as a nurse.

Drawing upon personal qualities and leadership skills are important aspects of improvement. Read about Sherry's improvement – Improving choice – to learn why.

Case study   Improving choice

Sherry was on placement in a residential setting for people with a learning disability. She really liked the homeliness of the place but noticed that it was very difficult to involve the people she was caring for in choosing what they would like for their meals, as many had great difficulty communicating. Though the staff tried very hard, Sherry thought there must be a way they could better support the residents with choosing their meals. She noticed that pictures worked well when communicating for other purposes, so she devised a picture-based version of the menu and tried using it one day with Paul, who she often worked with. Once she explained to him that she wanted him to choose what he wanted to eat from the pictures, his eyes lit up! She wouldn't necessarily have put together some of the foods he had in one meal – but it wasn't her lunch after all! This method worked so well for Paul that Sherry decided to try using it with other residents to see if it made things easier for them too – which it did – so before long, there were picture-based versions of the menu in regular use.

Chapter summary

The role of quality improvement in healthcare has evolved over the last three decades. This has been in response to many issues, but arguably most importantly where service users and those close to them were harmed by both individuals and organisations failing in their duty of care. This has resulted in quality improvement becoming a fundamentally important aspect of the role of all healthcare professionals, an approach to 'making healthcare safe, effective, service user-centred, timely, efficient and equitable' (THF, 2021, p7). Thus, quality improvement is a tool enabling nursing students and registered nurses to ensure that every service user, family and carer receives the best possible care. Further than this, it also ensures that health professionals themselves can influence practice and ensure they are working in the most effective manner.

Quality improvement involves working in partnership with a wide range of others, service users, their families, carers and other staff to name but a few, to add value to the care delivered. Developing an 'improvement mind-set' in respect of all actions we undertake is key. Working in this way, all nurses can undertake improvement as part of their normal everyday practice, constantly generating small innovations, which when combined result in improvement upon a grand scale.

Glossary

Contemporary: current, up to date
Human-centric: focus upon human beings
Innovation: something new and original that creates value
Key drivers: the reasons why change is needed

Answers to activities

Activity 1.3 Measuring

Figure 1.4 identifies some of the key stakeholders that Harry may need to consider along with one way of visually depicting a basic analysis of how involved they will need to be in any change. The closer they are to the inner circle represents how closely involved they will be. It is also worth considering that some stakeholders may have a lot of power or need to give permission for an improvement idea to be tested but then have limited, or intermittent involvement at specific stages, rather than be heavily involved throughout.

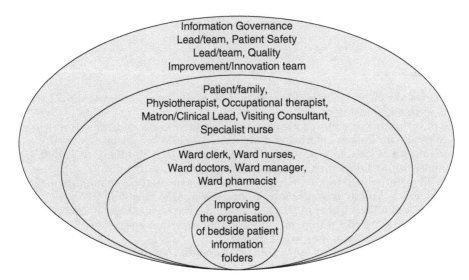

Figure 1.4   Identifying Harry's stakeholders

Activity 1.4 Reflection

My personal definition of innovation is

> *A change in the way I, or others work, which results in an increase in service user satisfaction with the care or services they receive.*

As we have discussed so far in the chapter, it can be difficult to find a definition that applies to all situations, but to my mind innovation means making an improvement for service users. In my practice I constantly question whether what I am doing is the best approach, and how satisfied the person or people receiving the care, or service, actually are.

As you read through the rest of the chapter, think further about your definition of innovation and mine, and see how they could be further improved.

Activity 1.7 Measuring

This is an example of an 'Astonishment Report' from somebody attending a General Practice in which people are asked to identify aspects of their experience of the service that astonish them in terms of being excellent or needing development.

Positives:

- A very warm welcome; engaging reception staff; smiling faces; passing staff noticed I wasn't sure how to use the 'booking in screen' and offered to help.
- Quality of the environment – clean and tidy waiting room, comfortable chairs and a variety of styles – some raised seats making it easier to get up, clear signs and notices in large letters.
- Children's area with good quality toys for different ages.
- 'WOW' moment – clinician was so patient and really made me feel like they were listening to me even though I know they had plenty of other people waiting.
- The receptionist anticipated my needs when I left the consultation room – and enquired whether I needed to book another appointment before I could ask – she must have noticed the slip of paper the nurse gave me in my hand! – excellent! – wish I had taken notice of their name.
- I was seen earlier than my appointment time – an added bonus – which meant I didn't have to wait long for the bus home.

Not so positives:

- No obvious way of letting anybody know I'd arrived for my appointment if I hadn't been able to work the 'booking in' machine.
- No adult seating in the children's area, caused me stress as my daughter wanted to play but I couldn't stand for long or get up and down from the child size chairs.
- Great selection of kids' toys but they didn't look very clean and there was nothing there to wipe them with, so I didn't really want my daughter to touch them.
- I was a bit overwhelmed by all the information – so many notices reminding me to 'do this' or 'check that' – I try to look after myself but it was just too much!
- The monitor to tell me where to go when it was my turn was quite small and I couldn't really see it, so I was worried I'd miss my appointment – and my name wasn't called so I don't know how people who can't see would manage.
- It took me six weeks to get my appointment – I couldn't get through on the telephone and I haven't been able to work the online booking system since I registered there.

Further reading

Ham, C, Berwick, D and Dixon, J (2016) *Improving Quality in the English NHS: A Strategy for Action.* London: The Kings Fund.

Excellent summary of key policy reforms that have driven quality improvement in the UK and the introduction and subsequent disbandment of key national bodies designed to drive and support improvement.

NHS England (n.d.) *Improvement Leaders Guides.* Coventry: NHS Institute of Innovation and Improvement, available at https://bit.ly/3u2vYkb

Series of 15 easy-read mini-guides covering three themes: General Improvement Skills, Process and Systems Thinking and Personal and Organisational Development. Each contains practical improvement tools, exercises and real examples of application in practice.

NHS Improving Quality (2014) *First Steps towards Quality Improvement: A Simple Guide to Improving Services,* available at: https://bit.ly/3NqDyvA

Contains the key information needed to undertake a successful quality improvement project. Includes the most relevant tools with other resources signposted for further exploration.

Useful websites

https://www.england.nhs.uk/patient-safety/ NHS Patient Safety – resources to support prevention of unintended consequences or harm during healthcare.

http://www.ihi.org/ Institute of Healthcare Improvement (USA) – resources and training to support the use of Improvement Science to enhance health and social care outcomes.

https://www.improvementacademy.org/ Improvement Academy – work with healthcare services, people accessing services and the public to deliver practical, tried and tested theory-based approaches to improvement.

http://www.patientvoices.org.uk/ Patient voices – reflective digital storytelling of healthcare experiences to provide insight and drive organisational change and growth.

https://www.thisinstitute.cam.ac.uk/ THIS.Institute (The Healthcare Improvement Studies Institute) – resources to support creating an evidence base that supports replicable and scalable improvements.

Chapter 2

Understanding the principles of quality improvement and your own contribution

Gillian Janes and Jill Foley

NMC Future Nurse: Standards of Proficiency for Registered Nurses

This chapter will address the following platforms and proficiencies:

Platform 5: Leading and managing care and working in teams

5.1 understand the principles of effective leadership, management, group and organisational dynamics and culture and apply these to team working and decision-making.

Platform 6: Improving safety and quality of care

6.4 demonstrate an understanding of the principles of improvement methodologies, participate in all stages of audit activity and identify appropriate quality improvement strategies.

6.9 work with people, their families, carers and colleagues to develop effective improvement strategies for quality and safety, sharing feedback and learning from positive outcomes and experiences, mistakes and adverse outcomes and experiences.

Platform 7: Co-ordinating care

7.13 demonstrate an understanding of the importance of exercising political awareness throughout their career, to maximise the influence and effect of registered nursing on quality of care, patient safety and cost effectiveness.

Chapter aims

After reading this chapter you should be able to:

- demonstrate an understanding of key improvement methods and tools;
- discuss how to apply these to support a systems approach to improvement within the context of your practice;
- identify your own contribution to improvement;
- explore the importance of engaging with key stakeholders for improvement;
- develop a greater awareness of your own quality improvement capability and use relevant resources to support your development as an improver.

I've seen some things that surprise me but what do I know about how to improve things – I'm only just getting to grips with being a nurse and a useful part of the team.

(Lucy, 2nd year student nurse)

I've tried to make improvements in the past which I know would make things better for people but it was a waste of effort – everybody agreed with my suggestion but when I wasn't there they just did what they'd always done.

(Brian, registered nurse)

Introduction

Knowing what improvement is, why it is needed, and its relevance as a core part of the nurse's role is one thing; working out what that means for you as an individual is quite another. Maybe you see yourself as someone who can introduce and lead improvements to enhance people's care. Or perhaps right now you are feeling more like the colleagues quoted at the start of this chapter, busy focusing on delivering good quality nursing care like Lucy; or disillusioned by the limited success of previous improvement attempts like Brian. This chapter will enable you to explore your current improvement capability and develop a focused plan for enhancing this. It will also help you develop your understanding of core improvement principles such as systems thinking, co-production and leadership; along with commonly used improvement tools.

Activity 2.1 will help you establish your improvement baseline. Your responses should provide clues to your strengths and areas to explore further to help develop your improvement expertise. Record your responses for use later in this chapter.

Activity 2.1   Reflection

Reflect upon your improvement knowledge, role, skills and confidence. Use the questions below to focus your thinking and remember there is no correct answer.

Do you feel able to improve nursing/healthcare practice and lead improvement initiatives?

- Yes
- No
- Not sure

How confident do you feel about sharing your improvement ideas and leading improvement?

- Very
- Moderately
- Somewhat
- Not confident

Reflect upon:

- Why you answered this way
- What else you need to know or do to become more confident about being involved in improvement activity
- Whether you see yourself as a leader?
  - Yes
  - No
  - Not sure

As we have seen in previous chapters, successful improvement can be complex, drawing on knowledge and practice from many disciplines. This can make knowing where to start when you have an improvement idea overwhelming. To help overcome this by developing your knowledge of Improvement Science, we focus on a small selection of evidence-based approaches that are commonly used and potentially most relevant to practitioner-based improvement.

Figure I.1 in the Foundations chapter illustrates that it can help to think about improvement in terms of three facets:

1. Core principles for healthcare improvement.
2. Methods and tools used to support the application of these principles in practice.
3. The personal knowledge and skills needed to effectively participate in or lead improvement.

This chapter examines each of these facets in more detail.

Exploring improvement principles methods and tools

Core improvement principles

Use systems thinking

Before embarking upon an improvement, it is important to have a good understanding of the quality issue you are focusing on, and the conditions that will maximise your chances of implementing successful change.

Even when the case for change is clear and the improvement idea seems simple, successfully introducing change in healthcare can often prove extremely difficult. Figures vary but at best improvement projects generally have a 50/50 chance of success; therefore, Brian's experience at the start of this chapter is common. Understanding the systems within which healthcare operates, however, can really improve the likelihood of success.

Healthcare is a complex adaptive system (CAS); other CAS examples include the immune system, an insect colony or a family. A CAS is defined as:

> *a dynamic network of agents acting in parallel, constantly reacting to what the other agents are doing, which in turn influences behaviour and the network as a whole.*

> (Holland, 1992)

Thus, focusing on recognising patterns and interrelationships rather than traditional linear causes and effects is important when trying to understand or achieve change in healthcare. A CAS is characterised by constant adaptation and is often embedded within other systems that interact and co-evolve (Plesk, 2003). Sustainable improvement therefore often requires a complex change intervention based on the application of contextual, technical and leadership expertise. Activity 2.2 will help you understand why this is so and what you can do to ensure the best chance of success.

Activity 2.2   Building knowledge

Watch these three-minute videos (Part 1 and 2) for an explanation of Edwards Deming's Theory of Profound Knowledge and the complex nature of change in healthcare.

- https://www.youtube.com/watch?v=mJSJzC43W10
- https://www.youtube.com/watch?v=TKdfGUehj20

As Deming's theory illustrates, leading or spreading healthcare improvement involves complex or so-called 'wicked problems'. The examples of baking a cake, sending a rocket to the moon and raising a child described by Glouberman and Zimmerman (2002) are often used to illustrate the difference between simple, complicated and complex issues (see Table 2.1).

Example	Problem type	Approach	Other factors	Outcome
Baking a cake	Simple	Follow a recipe, i.e. ingredients and method	Cooking skills helpful but not essential for success	Generalisable process and results lead to likely success
Sending a rocket to the moon	Complicated	Using formulaic and expert knowledge	Learn from unexpected events to enhance future success by building improvements into the system	Fairly predictable – rockets are similar in important ways so success with one gives reasonable chance of success with another
Raising a child	Complex	Expert advice and past experience is only a starting point	Interaction between the subject and approach Unpredictable response	Applying a previously successful formula does not necessarily lead to the same outcome and may itself have a negative effect, e.g. if the child resents being treated the same as someone else

Table 2.1 Summary of simple, complicated and complex problems

Thinking back to Harry's situation and difficulty finding the observation chart in the overcrowded records, what type of problem do you think this is? At first glance it might seem simple and easily resolved by reorganising the files, perhaps using colour coding so everyone can find what they need. But what order should the documents be filed in? The nurses and doctors may think the observation chart should be first, whereas the pharmacists could want the prescription chart to take precedence, the physiotherapist may be most interested in how well the person has been mobilising so may think this information should come before the prescription chart, and the patient or family may have their own priorities. These are just examples of the different groups, functions or parts of the complex system within which the bedside records are embedded, but may explain why Harry's assessor suggested his first step was to identify the stakeholders who might need to be involved in his project. Perhaps the assessor recognised that what seems like a simple improvement idea requires collaborative leadership to enhance Harry's chances of success, as numerous individuals and groups use the records for interrelated but often quite different purposes. We return to collaborative, or collective leadership for improvement later in this chapter.

Design for humans: use Human Factors science

The complex work processes healthcare involves remain predominantly human centric and therefore prone to the intrinsic fallibility of humans. Though progress is being made, healthcare lags years behind other high-risk industries including nuclear, airline, rail, and oil and gas production in recognising the importance of designing work systems that account for human fallibility in attempting to reduce errors and promote staff wellbeing. Human Factors (or Ergonomics) focuses on:

rigorous, elegant, evidence-based solutions to problems and building resilient systems that enable people to do the right things, every time.

(CIEHF, 2019, p2)

The discipline of Human Factors is concerned with the dynamic interaction between the task and the environment in which it takes place. This includes, for example, other members of the team, the design of equipment and work processes, and individual human characteristics. The aim is to make it easy to do the right thing. A short animation explains Human Factors principles and their application in healthcare (see the further reading section at the end of this chapter).

Reviewing Harry's example, we see that the bedside records folder is a form of 'equipment', used to support the care process that a range of healthcare staff interact with. Taking Harry's situation a step further, the records are only one small part of wider care delivery processes; therefore it is important that any potential improvement effort involves the application of Human Factors principles to maximise success. Additional resources at the end of this chapter will help you develop a more in-depth understanding of this topic.

Be scientific and systematic

Improvement Science is about finding out how to improve and make changes in the most effective way. It is about systematically examining the methods and factors that best work to facilitate quality improvement.

(The Health Foundation, 2011, p3)

As outlined in the Foundations chapter, Figure F1, Improvement Science is an overarching framework within which sit the Discipline of Improvement and the core principles underpinning it.

The terms *Improvement* Science and *Implementation* Science are sometimes used interchangeably so can easily be confused; they are different, however. Improvement Science draws on approaches from non-healthcare, high risk and process industries to support pragmatic reduction of poor healthcare performance and can be viewed as the overarching umbrella for improving services. Implementation Science arises from behavioural science and has a narrower focus on implementing new evidence into practice. Although these complementary disciplines arise from different philosophical perspectives and still operate relatively separately, they also overlap as both are used to support approaches to making things better. The 'science' element is also shared and refers to using a systematic planned approach, which can be replicated, measured and tested by collecting evidence to demonstrate if and/or how an improvement occurred.

Various improvement methods are available, each with its own limitations, but all are designed to support a systematic approach. They do this by prompting consideration, in a comprehensive and ordered manner, of all the relevant factors that might impact upon choosing which improvement to make and its likely success; this minimises the risk of missing something important.

Later chapters will explore change models in detail; however, it is important to note here that improvement is about developing ways to change things for the better. Thus change is an important element within improvement frameworks such as the MFI, which enable it to be applied in a structured and planned manner.

Plan for improvement

Strategic project management will help ensure a systematic and well organised improvement approach. From the outset, the overall purpose of the improvement must be clearly defined and key stakeholders identified. Developing **Terms of Reference** and a detailed management plan with stakeholders enables everyone involved to understand the scope of the improvement, their roles and time frames. A Gantt chart is commonly used to plot a schedule at this stage by identifying each activity against a timeline.

Jointly developing detailed aims, the project plan, the improvement methods and interventions to be used and how they will be tested also helps ensure that the improvement meets all stakeholder needs. Using a recognised strategic framework like the six domains of healthcare system quality (safe, effective, patient centred, timely, efficient and equitable quality (Institute of Medicine Report, 2001) or TEPEES (Timely, Effective, Person-centred, Efficient, Equitable, Safe) (The Health Foundation, 2013) introduced in Chapter 1 can help the team frame how the problem and overall aims are defined and fit with the wider context.

Use appropriate improvement methods and tools

A variety of tools and techniques are available to support each stage of the improvement process. For example, at the initial stage the problem being addressed needs to be clearly understood; Part 1 of the MFI asks *What are we trying to accomplish?* To answer this question, tools to facilitate the examination of cause and effect and interconnected relationships, e.g. Process or Value Stream Mapping Ishikawa (Fishbone diagram), Five Whys, and Lewin's Force Field Analysis are often used. Further information on a wide range of improvement tools can be found at: https://www.england. nhs.uk/quality-service-improvement-and-redesign-qsir-tools/ or https://learn.nes. nhs.scot/1262/quality-improvement-zone/qi-tools

Some tools are used in different ways at different project stages. For example, stakeholder identification is used during the initial stages to discover the key stakeholders, as we saw with Harry's idea and example in Chapter 1. Stakeholder analysis then explores the interests and priorities of those involved or affected by the proposed improvement or changes being introduced. This analysis informs the development of a stakeholder management and communication plan, which promotes effective continued engagement and communication about the improvement with everyone involved. It is very important that the needs of different stakeholders continue to be met as the project moves forward and the plan facilitates this. Later chapters (e.g. Chapter 4) will explore these improvement tools in further detail.

Use SMART

Commonly attributed to Peter Drucker, the SMART acronym (*Specific, Measurable, Attainable, Relevant and Time-bound*) is a tool that can be applied to each stage of the model to provide a clear focus. For example, when answering the initial three questions in Part 1 of the MFI it helps ensure the improvement team set clear criterion-based aims and outcome measures for the change, and it will do the same throughout the second stage of the model when the Plan Do Check Act (PDCA) cycles are implemented.

Measure and evaluate

Once clear aims have been established the measurements that will be used to test whether they are achieved, and the changes designed to make the improvement, are identified. Using a combination of measurement tools to test these changes, and generate quantitative and qualitative data from which to draw conclusions, will help ensure the efficacy, efficiency and effectiveness of the proposed changes that are considered in terms of whether they work and why. Measures should include structure, process and outcome measures (Donabedian, 2005); and balancing measures to test that the changes designed to improve one part of the system are not causing new problems elsewhere (NHSE&I, 2018).

Evaluating the changes being tested against the project aim(s) through accurate measurement is extremely important. Choosing appropriate measures and data collection tools that are easy to use, provide information that accurately measures the change and its impact and produce data that can be analysed and interpreted quickly, helps facilitate the change process and determine whether the change results in actual improvement. Different types of measurement tools are available, including some with which you will be familiar. Audit, for instance, can establish the current situation or baseline. Re-auditing after each change cycle will provide comparative information to help determine each cycle's impact.

Most successful improvements use between three and eight measures and measurement tools, each providing different types of information, to enable an understanding of all aspects of the project (Healthcare Improvement Scotland, 2017). For example, a change in waiting times can be measured numerically as a percentage, while rating scales and surveys can measure and explore people's satisfaction or perceptions. Whatever the tool used, it is of fundamental importance that it is appropriate for the relevant measurement criteria, and these criteria reflect the corresponding project aim/s. For example, if the aim is to achieve 100% adherence to a procedure and the measurement tool is observational audit, the audit criteria must accurately reflect the procedure and not be open to interpretation by individual observers.

During the implementation stage, measurement data can be collected and plotted on a timeline to support ongoing analysis. This approach helps identify patterns and trends from which to draw conclusions and make decisions. A run chart is a tool commonly used for this purpose, to support the visualisation of results over time and in relation to contextual issues such as the introduction of each new PDCA cycle. A temperature, pulse and respiration (TPR) chart is a good example of a run chart you will be familiar with. Tools used to help identify patterns for potential intervention based on similar principles are found across health and social care contexts. For instance, you will probably have seen numerous run charts illustrating changing Covid-19 rates and related hospital admissions, with interventions such as vaccine availability and immunisation uptake statistics highlighted to help illustrate key dates and the impact of interventions.

Measuring for improvement may seem complicated, but do not be put off. Using measurement tools and data to monitor and evaluate clinical parameters is a core nursing skill you are developing so you already have relevant transferable skills to apply to this aspect of improvement practice. Measuring improvement will be explored further in Chapters 5 and 6.

Lead for improvement

Improvement does not happen without purposeful consideration and action, which often demands leadership. Leadership is a dynamic concept commonly referred to as an art and a science; an art because the qualities and skills it entails cannot just be learned from a textbook, and a science because of the growing body of knowledge regarding the leadership process, skills involved and their application in practice. Leadership theory continues to evolve and is detailed elsewhere (see the further reading section at the end of this chapter). Theory development is contextual, however, and because compassionate, inclusive and collective leadership is central to delivering high-quality care and the staff support and positive cultural change required to achieve this (Oxlade, 2020), it will be our focus.

As we saw earlier, in complex adaptive systems like healthcare, which involve dynamic interactions between evolving elements and sub-systems comprising multiple individuals and groups, relational, adaptive and engaging leadership is necessary for success. Thus role-modelling and facilitating the adoption of a collective leadership approach is necessary (James, 2011) to promote and embed an improvement culture. The Chief Nursing Officer (CNO) for England's statement below illustrates what this means in practice:

Collective leadership is about everyone taking responsibility not just for their own job or role, but for the success of their team and... organisation as a whole. It is about ensuring that all voices are valued and contribute to the conversations where decisions are made.

(https://www.england.nhs.uk/nursingmidwifery/shared-governance-and-collective-leadership/)

In requiring everyone takes responsibility for the success of the organisation rather than just their own job or work area, collective leadership firmly situates leadership as an emergent event rather than a person or role. This reflects the distributed leadership approach described by Gronn (2000), which enables leadership to emerge from a collective social process involving the interactions of multiple individuals. Such leadership is associated with relatively 'flat' organisational structures and an inclusive learning culture rather than the top-down approaches linked to a rigid hierarchy. The 'snowflake model' of community organising leadership, first described by Marshall Ganz and now used by the influential Institute for Healthcare Improvement (IHI), provides an example of this approach – see: CL Toolkit ChapterLeadershipStructure.pdf (ihi.org). Thus, not only is improvement 'everybody's business' but now we learn that, according to contemporary theory, so too is leadership. This may surprise you, as it contrasts with previous leadership approaches, which have traditionally focused on developing individual capability without recognising the need to develop the collective or embed leader development within the person's work or organisational context.

Collective leadership cultures are characterised by all staff focusing on continual learning and, through this, on the improvement of outcomes and services. It requires high levels of dialogue, debate and discussion to achieve shared understanding about quality problems and solutions. It is argued that this can only be achieved through compassionate leadership as a lack of compassion has been identified as a key contributory factor in numerous healthcare scandals and failures in care delivery. For example, the Kings Fund (2020) Courage of Compassion Report highlighted the proven link between staff wellbeing and high-quality care, and the role of compassionate leaders in addressing the three core needs of nurses and midwives for autonomy, belonging and contribution if they are to flourish and thrive at work.

Compassionate leadership comprises four elements (West, 2021):

- Attending: being present, listening and noticing others' suffering.
- Understanding: the others' situation through a listening dialogue and balanced appraisal of the cause to achieve shared understanding.

- Empathising: mirroring the other's feelings, without being overwhelmed or needing to solve or intervene.
- Helping: taking thoughtful, wise and appropriate action based on what is most useful to others.

As with the transformational leadership theory that went before it, however, compassionate leadership does not involve compromising commitment to good performance management, having difficult conversations, or being able to challenge the status quo. Rather, it creates a culture of learning, encourages risk-taking (within boundaries) and an acceptance that not all improvement ideas will succeed. Together these create psychological safety for staff who can then feel confident about speaking out and trying out ideas for better ways of delivering services (RCN, 2021).

Build an improvement culture

An improvement culture embraces continuous learning and change to improve quality. Key elements of developing an improvement culture are creating psychological safety and applying the principles of collective and compassionate leadership. West et al (2017) describes how a culture shaped by compassion is a fundamental enabling factor for improvement and innovation:

> *Compassion ... creates psychological safety, such that staff feel confident in speaking out about errors, problems and uncertainties and feel empowered and supported to develop and implement ideas for new and improved ways of delivering services.*

> (West et al, 2017, p2)

An organisation's culture may be defined as 'the way things are done around here' and is driven by a set of shared values or assumptions. Often these values and assumptions and how they impact upon aspects of practice are hidden and may not always reflect what is publicly advocated. Because culture influences how people within the organisation behave, it is not enough to say 'these are our values, and they guide what we do' – organisations, teams and individuals must live those values day to day and be seen to be doing so. Understanding the existing culture and why "things are done this way" is fundamental when introducing change and trying to make improvements. It is also important to appreciate that a number of different subcultures may exist within organisations and teams.

Senior leaders, in positions of power, have a crucial role in developing an improvement culture. However, we all contribute to the culture in which we work through our words, actions and behaviour. For example, in the illustration at the start of this chapter, Brian mentions colleagues agreeing to changes, then reverting back to what they have always done. There are many reasons why this can happen. Lack of self-confidence and knowledge may mean the potential change causes anxiety and takes people out of their comfort zone. How the change is introduced may also be a factor. For instance, Brian says he 'knows the change would make things better' – but did he ask his colleagues for their views and help?

A shared vision and sense of ownership is fundamental to successful change, and role-modelling a collective leadership approach in which we are seen to value everyone's contribution is one means by which we can all help shape the prevailing culture. Perhaps Brian's colleagues had reservations about the change but felt unable to say what they really thought, so did not engage with it. Or perhaps they had tried to make changes but had not been supported, which affected their response to Brian's improvement, but he was unaware of this because 'he didn't ask'. Whatever the reasons, Brian's intentions are good though the experience appears to have left him feeling deflated, having wasted what he perceives as time and effort and perhaps reluctant to put improvement ideas forward in the future. Applying the principles of compassionate leadership and change theory to Brian's example may have helped create a culture within which more open and constructive dialogue could take place. This in turn may help the generation and implementation of improvement ideas more successfully in the future.

The Kings Fund explored how a culture of improvement can be embedded in an organisation with senior NHS leaders and key stakeholders (Jabbal 2017). They identified supportive factors including:

- leadership that moves away from top-down imposition and approaches;
- recognising that teams, service users and carers are often able to develop solutions to improvement problems because of their experiences;
- allocating adequate financial and human resources and time, and therefore demonstrating commitment to improvement;
- celebrating success; and
- placing service users and carers at the centre of improvement strategies.

Activity 2.3 will help you understand some of the approaches used in your organisation.

Activity 2.3   Critical thinking

1. Read your organisation's and department's mission statement/philosophy:
   a. What do they say about valuing people, leadership and improvement?
   b. Do these statements complement each other?
   c. How in your experience are they reflected in practice?
   d. How do policies and procedures reinforce the mission statements' values?
2. How are staff at all levels encouraged and supported to develop their leadership and improvement knowledge and skills? For example, through education, training and mentorship.
3. How do staff, service users and carers provide feedback regarding their experiences and make suggestions for improvement? What is done with this information?
4. How are staff and service users and carers engaged in improvement initiatives?
5. How is staff resilience supported?

Ensuring organisational systems and processes are inclusive, compassionate and appropriately supportive contributes to psychological safety and helps build resilience. This benefits staff wellbeing and promotes an improvement culture and safer care.

Activity 2.3 includes a question about staff resilience because it is recognised that resilience helps people cope with the demands placed upon them. Within the context of improvement, coping with continuous change in addition to the inherently physically and psychologically challenging nature of healthcare work can be very demanding. Strategies aimed at individuals to help them develop resilience by, for example, 'switching off' at the end of the working day and focusing on how to develop self-care and a healthy work–life balance, are promoted across the literature and within organisations. There is increasing recognition, however, that organisations also have responsibility for enabling a resilient workforce. This includes identifying and addressing inadequacies in the design of work systems that do not account for inherent human fallibility and taking account of other contextual factors outside the control of individual staff (Janes et al, 2022). For example, while still recognising the need for accountability in terms of errors and near misses, there has been a move away from punitive to learning approaches. By exploring why errors or near misses occur using systematic procedures such as root cause analysis, organisations can better understand contextual factors as well as those relating to the individuals involved. To have maximum effect it is important that the prevailing culture within which such tools are used is focused on learning rather than blame. For example, the impact of specific work patterns on fatigue and the associated increased risk of error is well documented. Though a delicate balance needs to be struck between service needs and staff wellbeing, organisations adopting a supportive learning and improvement culture are more likely to attract and retain staff and deliver high quality care. This type of working environment also encourages openness, honesty and transparency when things go wrong; this is an expectation of the NMC Code (2018b) and the professional duty of candour. Data collected through incident reporting and risk assessments can then be used to instigate or inform improvement activities.

Co-produce by engaging others in improvement

Key components of successful improvement initiatives and cultures include valuing people, engagement and recognising that improvement ideas and solutions can come from anyone who has experience of using services or working in an organisation. This can include people accessing services, their carers or advocates and healthcare staff, including non-clinical staff. A very effective example of this is the #hellomynameis campaign. Led by Dr Kate Granger and based on her experience of receiving healthcare as a person with terminal cancer, her very simple idea still has worldwide impact today.

Co-production characterises an inclusive approach to generating and managing change; it is underpinned by partnership working, which recognises and breaks down power differentials. The NMC (2018a), in their Standards Framework for Nursing and Midwifery Education (SFNME), define 'co-produced' as:

when an individual influences the support and services received, or when groups of people get together to influence the way that services are designed, commissioned and delivered, acknowledging that people who use social care and health services (and their families) have knowledge and experience that can be used to make services better. Co-production is one of the principles of the Care Act (2014).

(p13)

Co-production has a number of key principles including equality, diversity, access and reciprocity (SCIE, 2015). Activity 2.4 will help develop your understanding of co-production, its underpinning values and how to apply them to your improvement practice. These videos, produced by the Social Care Institute for Excellence (SCIE), explore what co-production means and how it differs from participation.

Activity 2.4   Building knowledge

Watch these videos (Part 1, 2 and 3) for an explanation of co-production. They explore the concept within the context of social care, but the principles apply across different sectors.

Co-production at SCIE and beyond part 1 and 2

- https://www.youtube.com/watch?v=D0lQsYZy9mo&list=PLxXjtx4-ZkqKcUBlKB2kiwV-opn9MZa7A&index=1
- https://www.youtube.com/watch?v=19IrSBC7GJA&list=PLxXjtx4-ZkqKcUBlKB2kiwV-opn9MZa7A&index=2

What makes co-production different from participation?

- https://www.youtube.com/watch?v=iJjmFYSB_qo&list=PLxXjtx4-ZkqKcUBlKB2kiwV-opn9MZa7A&index=3

Co-production is an important element of Improvement Science and nursing; for example, the NMC Future Nurse standards (NMC, 2018a) were co-produced. The quotation below is taken from *Enabling Professionalism* (NMC, 2018b), which was commissioned by the CNOs for England, Wales, Scotland and Northern Ireland. It illustrates the scope of nursing practice within the context of improvement, and how nurses can influence and facilitate strategic and operational change.

Nurses and midwives play a critical role in strategy, service redesign and improving health outcomes, actively enabling co-production and decision making at all levels of policy making and service provision.

(Enabling Professionalism, NMC, 2018b, p3).

Here we see nursing actions as conduits for quality outcomes. Make a few notes identifying how you can facilitate co-production in your practice.

When completing Activity 2.3 you may have come across examples of how stakeholder feedback is gained and used to initiate improvement projects within your organisation. For example, the friends and family test (https://www.england.nhs.uk/fft/), 15 steps challenge (NHS England, 2017), staff surveys, leadership walk-arounds, improvement champions and service user/carer groups. How data is collected using these methods can be critiqued. For example, if you are asked your opinion during a healthcare experience you may not feel well enough to engage or be reluctant to offer less than satisfactory feedback as you are still receiving care. A halo effect is also recognised as people exit services. How and when you collect data is an important consideration when you select your evaluation methods.

A lot of service user feedback is collected by healthcare providers. The below case study outlines some of the findings of a study examining how patient experience data is used by frontline staff, and the role of team composition and diversity in improvement work.

Case study   Using service user experience data for improvement

Locock et al (2021) explored how ward teams in six sites used patient feedback to improve the patient experience. They found involving a range of professionals with different levels of seniority, and gaining support from patient experience teams, helped overcome some of the difficulties faced when taking improvements forward. This was because the more diverse teams were able to draw on different skills sets, resources and authority than those from single disciplines. They found that although the teams were encouraged to involve service users, their direct involvement was minimal. They suggest that service user involvement would enhance team creativity and the resources from which they can draw upon.

The values underpinning co-production and definitions we have seen emphasise that stakeholder involvement, where relevant, should be integral to each stage of the improvement process. As a general principle, project teams focusing upon person-centred improvements should include service users, carers and representatives from the inter-disciplinary groups who contribute to the aspect of care being considered. Each person's role and contribution should be valued equally, clearly defined and understood from the beginning of the project. Even when an improvement idea focuses on staff or a process service users may not be directly aware of, their input should be considered as they can provide appropriate insights. Embedding co-production can be difficult; however, the core nursing skills you are developing through involving and working with others are highly transferable to the improvement-related aspects of your practice. HQIP (2017) provides a comprehensive guide for how to involve service users and the public in improvement, including examples of best practice.

Ideally, you now recognise the importance of a collective, compassionate leadership approach and an inclusive learning culture for enabling co-production. This includes putting in place systems that encourage and are responsive to feedback. Also important is establishing and using effective listening and communication networks and infrastructures that clearly set out improvement roles, processes and related responsibilities. These principles are relevant at organisation and system level but can also be applied in your own practice, regardless of your role or level of responsibility. In this way you can role-model an inclusive learning approach; for example, listening to and involving service users and your colleagues, and developing and using the relevant structure to support the joint effort. This in turn enables you to influence the quality of care and prevailing organisational culture. Chapters 3 to 5 examine the principles of co-production further.

Exploring your own contribution to quality improvement

SCIE (2015) suggest that co-production can help build stronger communities and develop citizenship; thus it is a motivator for change as it encourages, values and supports involvement.

Professional and organisational citizenship

You may be very used to thinking of yourself as a citizen of your country, but have you ever thought about yourself as a professional citizen? A professional citizen actively participates in their profession by thinking about and trying to influence its future. In contrast, a professional inhabitant accepts the way things are and believes others are acting on their behalf (Fulton, 2019).

As we have seen, nurses have a professional responsibility to instigate, lead and actively participate in improvement. Professional citizens go a step further by actively seeking out opportunities to influence, help build and shape nursing. In contrast, professional inhabitants, although fulfilling threshold professional role requirements, which can themselves be very challenging, have not taken the next step and have not become a force for change. There are many opportunities for professional citizenship in nursing and healthcare; examples include being a course representative, and participation in peer support groups and national forums. Such activities are mechanisms for developing and presenting the collective voice of nursing and exerting influence; goals that nurse leaders and professional bodies promote through visioning and workstreams. For example, the CNO for England's vision sees nurses and midwives being listened to in 'all decision-making conversations'.

a collective voice can drive forwards transformation across health and care sectors and organisational boundaries. To achieve this staff must be supported to recognise and embrace that they are all leaders – no matter where you work, or the role that you have.

(Ruth May – https://www.england.nhs.uk/nursingmidwifery/shared-governance-and-collective-leadership/)

The below case study provides an example of professional citizenship.

Case study   New registrants and professional citizenship

The Royal College of Nursing (RCN) Newly Registered Nurse Network was launched on Twitter in June 2020 (#RCNNRN) to:

add the unique perspective of the newly qualified to the voice of nursing …

#RCNNRN provides peer support for students in the last six months of their nursing degree and registered nurses in the first 18 months of their careers. It is run by newly registered nurses and students; access at: https://www.rcn.org.uk/get-involved/forums/nrn-network

---

Citizenship can also be applied within an organisational context. Here, employees, by engaging and helping to shape how the organisation operates, contribute to its future rather than just turning up to work. Organisational and professional citizenship are key qualities employers look for in their workforce. However, the proposition that everyone has a leadership role, has a responsibility to improve the quality of the service they deliver and can influence wider healthcare practice no matter where they are placed within an organisation, may not be as straightforward as it seems. Complete activity 2.5 to examine how you might help Lucy explore her improvement role and citizenship in your practice.

Activity 2.5   Reflection

Looking back to Lucy's comments at the beginning of this chapter, the idea of citizenship and her role in improvement may not be something she would relate to:

I've seen some things that surprise me but what do I know about how to improve things – I'm only just getting to grips with being a nurse and a useful part of the team.

(Lucy, 2nd Year Student Nurse)

1. If you were helping Lucy reflect upon her improvement role, what would you say to her?

---

2.   How do you/could you contribute to your profession, the success of your team and the organisation within which you work?

There are numerous potential responses to these questions. Jot down your answers and refer to them as you complete Activity 2.6.

Nurse as QI participant, instigator and leader of change

You may have found Activity 2.5 quite difficult, and improvement may still seem a complex undertaking. Activity 2.6 provides some practice examples to help you explore improvement and citizenship further. Compare your responses with the debrief notes following the activity and your responses to Activity 2.5 to help cement your understanding of how these two elements of the nurse's role interact.

Activity 2.6   Reflection

Consider the following aspects of practice and reflect upon whether they can be described as improvement initiatives and/or examples of professional or organisational citizenship:

1.   Student nurse Sally attends a board meeting following an open invitation from the chair, who wants to hear about people's experiences of a new service. Sally shares her experience of working with the new integrated team.
2.   The NMC asks people to complete a survey exploring the Standards for education and training. Registrants and students from a ward team send a joint response, working through each question together before uploading it.
3.   A service user's abdominal wound is producing a lot of exudate. During consecutive nights the dressing leaks. Their named nurse Sam wants to find an alternative dressing. They ask the wound care nurse to visit and together with the service user they amend the care pathway. Sam explains how the new dressing works to colleagues during the evening huddle. Overnight a small amount of leakage occurs. The service user asks Sam to alter the normal timing of the dressing to later in the day. This is incorporated into the care plan. The dressing remains intact overnight.
4.   Eugene asks to take part in an audit of staff compliance with hand hygiene procedures, then presents the findings to the multidisciplinary team. The team share ideas and develop an action plan to increase compliance.
5.   Jay volunteers to help produce an online information site for people using a healthcare environment and students allocated there. This involves working with people accessing the service, a practice educator, a governance lead and representatives from

(Continued)

(Continued)

the department team. Each person has specific responsibilities and six PDCA cycles are used to finalise the site information.

6. Sia works on a children's ward. One of the children tells her she was frightened in the night by "shadow monsters" searching the bins. Sia tries to provide reassurance and says she will sit with her to see what is happening. She also spends time during the night shift observing the environment. She notices that when people walk past the nurses' station shadows are projected against the walls and opening and closing the bins is noisy. She asks the charge nurse if the lamps can be repositioned and silent bins ordered. The charge nurse agrees and helps Sia complete the documentation required to fund new bins. Sia writes a short report for the senior nurse forum. She explains that she never realised how noisy a ward is until she closed her eyes and listened.

7. Jonah is a healthcare assistant responsible for facilitating a monthly team discussion entitled 'let's talk about quality'. He introduced this having been asked by a carer to explain what high quality care means to someone who is frightened by their loss of independence and needs help going to the toilet. Jonah asks the team to share experiential learning and feedback to improve service users', carers' and the team's experiences. Learning is disseminated via the department notice board and website. His award-winning initiative has led to numerous small-scale but high impact changes.

All these scenarios demonstrate active contribution to improvement processes. Some are more systematic in their approach. Jay for example has been part of a planning and implementation group that used multiple PDCA cycles to develop an end-product. Sam effectively used the nursing process, which is a systematic decision-making tool, working in partnership with the service user to improve their care and ensure their suggestions were implemented. Sia also listened to the service user and responded with empathy by exploring their personal experience using a solution-focused approach. Jonah reflected upon the carer's question and placed himself in the service user's shoes. Having done so he used his experience to focus the team, initiating regular conversations about quality.

It can be argued that the scenarios exemplify professional citizenship in everyday nursing practice. Jay and Eugene, however, volunteered; Sally responded to an open invitation from a chair who wanted to hear and listen to people's experiences. The ward team chose to respond to the consultation. Sia advocated for change and wrote about her experience, disseminating good practice. The charge nurse helped her apply for funding to improve the service and used this as a development activity. In taking these approaches they have all been proactive and contributed to organisational and professional citizenship.

The scenarios illustrate positive role-modelling by front-line staff and excellent examples of the positive influence and important contribution everyone can make, regardless of their position or level of responsibility. They demonstrate the nurse's improvement role in influencing micro and macro level change. For example, this could be through leading national policy and strategy development, or personal interactions that make a positive difference to individual service users, carers and colleagues on a daily basis. Both are of equal importance.

Establishing your current quality improvement capability

As established earlier in this chapter, achieving improvement in a healthcare setting requires the application of a combination of contextual, technical and leadership expertise. Previous sections have introduced you to contextual and technical issues such as complexity and healthcare as a Complex Adaptive System. The Model for Improvement (MFI) has also been identified as one of the methods commonly used to guide small-scale, practitioner-based improvement. The remainder of this chapter will focus on helping you consider your current capability as an improver and formulating a personal action plan to develop this further.

Review your answers to Activity 2.1. Has your thinking changed, having considered the material in this chapter so far? If so, how and why do you think this is?

Personal development is a lifelong journey. Where you are on this journey will depend upon many factors, including previous experience, context and access to learning support. For example, you may or may not have been previously involved in improvement. It is also important, however, to consider the wider transferable skills you are continuing to develop during your nursing programme; for example, the interpersonal, team-working, problem-solving, decision-making and information management skills required for successful improvement.

There are many tools to support your development as a quality improver. We will use Figure F1 from the Foundations chapter as a general guide, plus the Healthcare Leadership Model (NHS Leadership Academy 2013) and reflective, self-assessment activities. The key focus of this section is on your leadership capability, as this enables the application of your more technical improvement knowledge and skills in practice. Subsequent chapters will explore how to apply the MFI in practice and how to lead others in more detail. The further reading section at the end of this chapter also provides information.

Leadership qualities

Personal effectiveness

What all current leadership theory has in common is a recognition of the need to lead self before leading others. This is connected to notions of followership, i.e. who would want to follow you if you cannot lead yourself, and the ability to ethically influence others based on trust and authenticity. These principles require that you have a clear vision, i.e. know what the desired but also possible future is, and are able to communicate this vision and inspire others to share it, thus enabling and guiding collaborative action. Landsberg (2003) depicts leadership as a simple equation:

Vision x Inspiration = Momentum

You are therefore unlikely to be able to influence others to support an improvement idea if you are unable to demonstrate personal effectiveness. Getting to know yourself is the first step to personal effectiveness. Self-knowledge involves uncovering the real you by weeding out all the messages, images, beliefs and expectations that you have taken on, perhaps as a result of your upbringing or other influences, but that do not actually belong to you. The more self-knowledge you possess, the more self-aware you will become and the easier it will be to identify areas you may need to develop and strengths that you could maximise, to become more effective. Warren Bennis (1989, p56) identified four lessons of self-knowledge:

1. You are your own best teacher
2. Accept responsibility
3. You can learn anything you want to learn
4. Understanding comes from reflecting on your experience.

Lessons 1–3 particularly reflect the idea of individual or personal agency, which is the term used to describe a feeling of being in control of our thoughts, actions and their consequences.

You will be developing critical reflection skills as a core part of your nursing programme and these are equally applicable in developing your improvement expertise. For example, before taking forward any improvement idea it is essential you identify what knowledge, qualities and skills you already possess, and at which stages during the process you may have difficulties because you lack a particular skill or information. To illustrate this, if you have low self-confidence and do not like public speaking, you may need to devise strategies to increase your confidence so that you can effectively engage relevant colleagues and other stakeholders.

Self-assessment

This is an important means of increasing self-knowledge and self-awareness. It is important to adopt an honest and objective approach to gain most benefit as this enables you to set realistic parameters for development and capitalise on your interests, strengths, competencies and current abilities. There is a range of widely available tools specifically designed to support assessment of organisations' improvement capability and formal development programmes to support individual development, but no freely available tool to support assessment of individual improvement capability. The activities in this section will therefore use a combination of relevant resources. Information on further options is provided at the end of the chapter should you prefer.

Before progressing to complete your own improvement self-assessment, we will consider what Harry's might look like based on the improvement idea he identi-fied at the start of Part 1 and the stakeholders he identified in Chapter 1 that he would need to engage. Harry rates his behaviour against the summary definitions of the six Cs from *Compassion in Practice* (DH, 2012) and *Leading Change Adding Value* (NHS England, 2016) using a simple scale of 0–3. There are no right or wrong answers in this type of exercise so long as you can justify your ratings; for example, by using previous experiences or feedback from others to inform your responses. Harry's self-assessment might therefore look something like that in Table 2.2. Because we cannot speak to him directly, brief reflection notes illustrate how he arrived at his self-rating.

As you can see from Harry's reflections, he is completing the assessment from the perspective of his specific improvement capability and considering how the nursing knowledge and skills he is developing are transferable to the improvement aspects of his role. He has already started to identify some strengths, e.g. caring, compas-sion and communication and some of the skills he thinks he will need to develop further to help him progress his improvement idea. For example, he highlights needing more courage to speak up and engage with senior colleagues, that he has relatively limited knowledge of the organisation and needs to develop his networks, plus a specific lack of knowledge about how to deal with resistance. Such topics are addressed in the following chapters within the context of identifying, planning, implementing and evaluating an improvement idea, but first complete your own self-assessment.

Self-assessment activities

Complete the following activities based on your general experience of leading or being involved in improvement activities or, like Harry, on a specific improvement idea you want to take forward. The activities focus first on your leadership capability and second, your broader improvement knowledge and skills.

The Healthcare Leadership Model (HCLM) (NHS Leadership Academy, 2013) is designed to support staff working in any health and care setting to become better leaders. It illustrates the leadership behaviours expected of everyone working in healthcare and is relevant for all staff, whether directly involved with service users or not and regardless of whether they have formal leadership responsibility. The model consists of nine dimensions with personal qualities like self-awareness, self-confidence and self-control that are necessary for successful development in these nine dimensions embedded throughout. Assessment of your leadership skills can

6 Cs and summary definitions	Self-rating 0=never, 1=sometimes, 2=mostly, 3=always	Harry's reflection
Care: our care helps the individual person, is consistently right for them and improves the health of the whole community.	3	One of my strengths and probably what brought me into nursing. I always get positive feedback from assessors and service users about my caring attitude.
Compassion: care is given through relationships based on empathy, respect and dignity	3	This also comes easily to me. I may feel differently in future – I've worked with some people who aren't as compassionate as I think they should be – maybe it's because the constant pressure wears you down? I have no problems behaving ethically so far but I guess this might be more of a challenge as I progress. I'm also not sure how I'll convince other people to trust me enough to want to help with an improvement.
Competence: ability to understand an individual's health and social needs and the expertise, clinical and technical knowledge to deliver effective care and treatments based on research and evidence.	2	This is '2' because I am passing all my practice assessments, doing quite well on the programme and always get good feedback. However, I know very little about service improvement, I've not even heard of some things mentioned so far, so this could easily be a '1' for the improvement part of my role.
Communication: central to successful caring relationships and effective team working. Listening is as important as what we say and do. Communication is the key to a good workplace that benefits service users and staff.	3	I know I'm a good communicator and team member because I always get that feedback in university and on placement. I expect I'll be able to use these skills when I'm involved in improvement although the context will be different. I've heard of Emotional Intelligence and think communication is part of that, so if I learn more about it I could use my communication skills to even greater effect.

6 Cs and summary definitions	Self-rating 0=never, 1=sometimes, 2=mostly, 3=always	Harry's reflection
Courage: to do the right thing for those we care for, to speak up when we have concerns and to have the personal strength and vision to innovate and embrace new ways of working.	1	I know I need to be more courageous. I definitely see when things can be improved, or good practice isn't happening consistently, but I've never been the type of person who's first to speak up. I did raise the record folders issue with my assessor, though I can't imagine having the courage to speak to some of the stakeholders we identified – some are very senior and I wouldn't even have known most of them were there if my supervisor hadn't helped. I haven't really thought about the need to be politically aware before but I'm beginning to realise it's important. The example of Sally attending the board meeting! I know now it isn't enough to have a good improvement idea if there are other factors that mean we're unlikely to be able to take it forward at this particular time. It also bothers me that I won't be able to deal with people who don't agree with my ideas or attempts to improve things.
Commitment: to patients and populations. Builds on commitment to improve the care and experience of patients, to take action to make this a reality for all and meet the challenges ahead.	2	I nearly gave this a '3'. I'm totally committed to nursing but how much I can achieve is limited by my level of courage. I'm also still getting used to the fact that being a leader and helping to improve services as well as deliver them is part of every nurse's role – including students. I'm very motivated and quite good at maintaining this even when things get difficult; however, I'm not sure how to motivate others except by setting a good example with my own behaviour. I now know that's called role-modelling and is quite important, but I'm sure there are other ways of motivating others that I could learn more about to get better at this.

Table 2.2   Harry's self-assessment of his improvement capability using the six Cs framework

take various forms. Recent years have seen increasing use of 360° leadership assessment by clinical staff; however, the process requires skilled facilitation and often involves a cost. Information on a 'do-it-yourself' 360° tool is provided in the additional resources, however as self-assessment is also very effective, we focus on that here, using the HCLM.

This will enable a structured but comprehensive self-assessment of your leadership capability and the HCLM resource hub (https://www.leadershipacademy.nhs.uk/resources/healthcare-leadership-model/) provides access to a range of additional resources, including a section specifically for students. Complete Activity 2.7 to begin your leadership self-assessment.

Activity 2.7   Reflection

Step 1: Familiarise yourself with the HCLM by downloading and reading the overview at: https://www.leadershipacademy.nhs.uk/resources/healthcare-leadership-model/ . This document provides an overview of the model, brief information on the nine dimensions and what they consist of, how it should be used and the evidence underpinning it.

Step 2: Access the HCLM hub at: https://bit.ly/2NQ3IdW and follow the instructions to complete the self-assessment questionnaire. Adopt a realistic perspective when completing the self-ratings – remember even the most effective Chief Executive of the largest healthcare organisation does not need to demonstrate all the behaviours listed 100% of the time!

Upon completing the questionnaire, you will have access to a summary of your ratings.

Step 3: Reflect on these results, e.g. are they what you expected or not? What might they mean in terms of developing your improvement contribution? You may wish to discuss the process and results with a friend, supervisor or practice assessor/lecturer. Do they agree the assessment reflects the 'you' they see and why?

Keep a record of this activity to use later when creating your development plan.

As Figure F1 in the Foundations chapter illustrates, though leadership capability is a key component of improvement, there are others. It is important therefore to consider your current knowledge and skills against these other topic areas to provide a rounded self-assessment. Complete Activity 2.8 to do this.

Activity 2.8   Measuring

Review Figure F1. Consider each element of the model in turn and rank them in order of your current level of knowledge and skills. Many of these topics are relatively broad and high level so it can be helpful to identify specific sub-elements within them to help differentiate your assessment to ensure it accurately reflects your current capability. Use the template (Activity 2.8) in the Additional Resources section at the end of this chapter to complete your improvement capability self-assessment. Ideally do this in discussion with your lecturer, practice assessor or peers to help you arrive at an honest and realistic assessment.

A template to support you is given at the end of this chapter.

Developing a quality improvement skills personal development plan

While identifying your improvement–related strengths and areas for development is useful, this is not enough in itself to support further development; you need to create a personal action plan.

You may be very familiar with action planning, having previously worked with supervisors and assessors to draw up learning contracts or plans. You can draw on this experience here but will also need to use what you learned earlier about SMART objectives and the self-assessment activities completed in the previous section when devising your improvement skills personal development plan. This plan is not about addressing every aspect of your self-assessment, rather you should choose a maximum of two leadership and two improvement-based skills or qualities to focus on. It is important to remember this task is part of a lifelong journey in developing improvement expertise. Thinking particularly of the 'T' in SMART, we suggest basing your plan on a 3–6 month timescale as a guide but do discuss this with your practice assessor or personal tutor.

Any action plan should contain core elements:

- Objectives or goal statements – *What do I want to achieve?*
- Rationale statements – *What will be the benefits of achieving each objective?*
- Action steps – *What you will do to achieve each objective?*
- Evaluation criteria – *How will you know whether or not each objective has been achieved?*
- Timescale – *by when?*

Finalising a personal, behaviour-change focused, improvement skills-based action plan like this is a major achievement, as planning your own development is not easy, particularly when it involves an unfamiliar topic or skillset. Table 2.3 provides a sample plan with two objectives. The first focuses on developing greater self-confidence (a personal quality needed for effective leadership) and the second on how to use service user feedback to improve services, which has a more specific improvement skills focus. The more detailed and SMART the action plan is, the more effective it will be as a practical tool you can use to guide your development. Though this sample is a developed, quite detailed plan it is a general guide rather than fully comprehensive, i.e. the rationale could include additional benefits for each objective along with more action steps. Notice that each action step has its own evaluation criteria and timescale. You will also see that the action steps and completion date form a natural order, spaced over the three months; this is a SMARTer approach that is realistic and avoids leaving everything to the end.

Use the worked example (Table 2.3) as a template to develop your own SMART improvement capability development plan. Your objectives and plan for achieving them, however, should focus on the priority improvement and leadership skills identified during the self-assessment exercises you did earlier. As you develop the elements of your plan, pay particular attention to the 'R' element of SMART, to ensure they are 'realistic'. Personal development can involve changing deeply established habits, requiring repeated practice, which often takes months or years; so do not expect to achieve this type of personal behaviour change 100% of the time straight away. For example, for an objective 'to be more confident when sharing improvement ideas with senior colleagues', achieving this on 50% of occasions within a period of, say, six weeks would be much more realistic but still a stretching target and worthwhile achievement.

Any plan is of little use unless implemented, so share your draft plan with your practice assessor or personal tutor. They can help you ensure it is SMART and with putting it into practice by integrating with your wider professional development to maximise benefit.

Chapter summary

This chapter has introduced a range of improvement principles, commonly used methods and tools and their application in practice. We hope this has enhanced your understanding of the complex issues involved but also how you can contribute to improving service user, carer or staff outcomes within the context of your role. As the chapter highlights, you are not alone, and engaging others from the start will actually maximise the chances of success.

Balancing the technical and improvement-specific learning with the more generic, but equally relevant, transferable nursing skills you are developing is important. Hence, examples of

Objective	Rationale	Action steps	Evaluation criteria/ evidence of changed behaviour	Timescale	Achieved/not achieved
1. To develop self-confidence	To: • maximise my effectiveness in the role • enable service users to have confidence in the service provided • increase others' confidence in me • maintain my motivation • reduce personal worry and stress • increase my job satisfaction • enable ongoing development in my role	Self-assess self-confidence level using rating scale of 1–10 Read [insert author] on building self-confidence and identify 1 tip Try out one tip/strategy from reading	Self-ratings will increase by at least 2 scale points overall Reading completed and can name chosen tip Have two examples of when used new tip/strategy	Monthly (months 1–3) End month 1 End month 2	

(Continued)

Table 2.3 (Continued)

Objective	Rationale	Action steps	Evaluation criteria/ evidence of changed behaviour	Timescale	Achieved/not achieved
		Identify a self-confidence role-model	Able to name role-model	End month 1	
		Observe their behaviour, language, ways of thinking about things/approaching problems etc. and identify two ways in which they use confident language, behaviour or thinking to try out for yourself	Able to identify two examples of how you have tried out your language/behaviour	End month 2	
			Provide example of how your language/ behaviour/thinking has changed	End Month 3	
		Keep an achievements log	Minimum 2 achievements listed in log	Ad hoc as occur	
				Months 1–2	
			Minimum one example of when log was used to support self-confidence	End month 3	
		Seek fortnightly performance feedback from: • Practice assessor/ lecturer • 1–2 peers	A minimum of three examples of how feedback received has enhanced self-confidence	End of month 3	

Objective	Rationale	Action steps	Evaluation criteria/evidence of changed behaviour	Timescale	Achieved/not achieved
		Keep a reflective log on my self-confidence	A minimum of two examples from the log of when I have demonstrated enhanced self-confidence (*e.g. volunteering to take on a new task/project you haven't done before etc.*)	Ad hoc as situations occur but a minimum of monthly, months 1–3	
2. To enhance my ability to use service user feedback to enhance service delivery	• Visible demonstration of my values, i.e. that I value the service user perspective • Will enable me to be a better advocate • Will enhance the validity and credibility of improvement initiatives • Uses one of my strengths, i.e. ability to build rapport and communicate well with service users, to enhance services • Enables me to more effectively contribute to delivery of the service user involvement policy • … …	Read [*insert title of resource e.g. HQIP (2017) Involving service users in QI*]	Reading complete and have a summary of learning from it. Have 3 examples of how frontline staff have successfully used service user feedback to achieve service improvement	End month 1	

(Continued)

Table 2.3 (Continued)

Objective	Rationale	Action steps	Evaluation criteria/ evidence of changed behaviour	Timescale	Achieved/not achieved
		Keep a log of service user identified issues/good practice I come across as part of my normal role	Able to list a minimum of 3 examples from the log	Ad hoc, by end month 2	
		Find out how my department/organisation gathers service user feedback – informal and formal feedback	Can identify sources of service user feedback that are available in my department/ organisation and how to access these	End month 2	
		Find out how service user feedback is currently used to enhance services in my organisation by speaking to peers, practice assessor, dept or trust improvement team.	Can articulate mechanisms my organisation uses to enable service user feedback to inform service improvements	End month 3	
		Explore what support is available in my department/organisation for service improvement	Can identify 3 contacts for support in taking forward an improvement idea based on service user feedback	End month 3	

Table 2.3   Sample action plan

how and where knowledge and skills you are gaining as part of the wider nursing programme have been highlighted. A substantial part of this chapter has focused on enabling increased awareness and further development of your personal qualities and leadership capability with a particular focus on improving services. Most importantly, we hope this chapter has demonstrated that an improvement focus should and can permeate every aspect of nursing practice and helped you think about how you do and can make a difference to people's healthcare experience and outcomes.

Topics touched on here are addressed in more detail in later chapters to enable you to build on what you have learned. You may already have ideas about how you can or do contribute to improvement projects, influence the quality agenda and contribute as a professional citizen. The next chapter will build on this to help you consider the most effective way to work with others in leading change.

Glossary

Macro level: large-scale regional or national level initiatives, which may involve policy directives; for example target setting and national standards.
Micro level: small-scale individual or local level initiatives
Terms of Reference: used to support groups, e.g. project teams, committees, working together to accomplish a shared goal by promoting a common understanding among stakeholders by defining:

- vision, objectives, scope and deliverables (what is to be achieved);
- stakeholders, roles and responsibilities (who will take part);
- resource, financial and quality plans (how it will be achieved);
- work breakdown structure and schedule (when it will be achieved);
- criteria for success, risks and constraints.

Answers to activities

Improvement topic (add your own/delete topics as required)	**Self-rating of knowledge and skills** 0=none, 1=basic, 2=moderate, 3=proficient	**Reflective notes**
Involving users, carers and staff in improvement		
Process and systems thinking		
Personal and organisational development		

(Continued)

Table 2.4 (Continued)

Improvement topic (add your own/delete topics as required)	Self-rating of knowledge and skills 0=none, 1=basic, 2=moderate, 3=proficient	Reflective notes
Personal development		
Organisational development		
Developing an improvement culture		
Initiating, sustaining and spreading improvement		
Identifying and prioritising improvement ideas		
Creating a case for improvement, scoping and identifying SMART aims		
Initiating – planning an improvement		
Implementing an improvement		
Evaluating and sustaining an improvement		
Principles of improvement		
Using a systematic approach/improvement science		
Co-production and engaging others in improvement		
Measuring for improvement		
Tools and strategies – review https://www.england.nhs.uk/quality-service-improvement-and-redesign-qsir-tools/ or equivalent for a list of QI tools and populate the rows below with tools of relevance for you – some examples are provided		
The Model for Improvement		
Stakeholder identification and management tools		
Driver diagrams		
Cause and effect identification, e.g. Ishikawa		
Sustainability model		
Statistical Process Control		
Value stream mapping		
Theory and methods		
Change theory		
Statistics		
Systems theory		
Human Factors/Ergonomics		
Clinical Science		
Behaviour change theory		
Organisational psychology		
Sociology of organisations		

Table 2.4 Improvement capability self-assessment template to support Activity 2.8

Further reading

Ellis, P (2019) *Leadership, Management & Team Working in Nursing* (3rd ed.). London: Sage.

Provides a brief summary of leadership theory.

Fisher, M and Scott, M (2013) *Patient Safety and Managing Risk in Nursing* (TNP series). London: Sage – Human Factors section.

NHS Health Education England (n.d.) *Human Factors: A Quick Guide*, https://youtu.be/aGZz3w5Hy8Y

Northouse, PG (2018) *Leadership: Theory and Practice* (8th edn). London: Sage.

A more comprehensive overview of leadership theory.

The Health Foundation (2010) *Complex Adaptive Systems: Evidence scan.* London: The Health Foundation.

A systematic synopsis of the research evidence on complex adaptive thinking and its application in healthcare and other sectors.

The Kings Fund (2022) *How Does the NHS in England Work and How Is It Changing*, https://www.kingsfund.org.uk/audio-video/how-does-nhs-in-england-work

A short animation from The Kings Fund explaining how the NHS in England works.

Useful websites

https://www.hellomynameis.org.uk/ #hellomynameis website

Other 360° freely available self-assessment tools:

Leadership:

- **https://www.leadershipacademy.nhs.uk/resources/healthcare-leadership-model/** Healthcare Leadership Model and associated resources
- Wedderburn Tate (1999) Becoming a transformational leader – includes a useful 10 question do-it-yourself 360° assessment resource with instructions.
- **https://www.nwpgmd.nhs.uk/sites/default/files/resiliencequestionnaire.pdf** Resilience

Psychometric tests:

- **https://www.goodjob.io/the-5-best-free-online-personality-tests/** Commonly used tests including Myers Briggs Personality Inventory (MBTI), DISC, 'colours' and emotional intelligence
- **https://www.truity.com/test/enneagram-personality-test** Enneagram
- **https://openpsychometrics.org/tests/IPIP-BFFM/** Big 5 (OCEAN)

Human Factors resources:

- **https://www.rcn.org.uk/clinical-topics/patient-safety-and-human-factors** RCN
- **https://chfg.org/** Clinical Human Factors Group: charity working to make healthcare safer. Established by Martin Bromiley after the death of his wife Elaine following a routine operation
- **https://www.england.nhs.uk/wp-content/uploads/2013/11/nqb-hum-fact-concord.pdf** Human Factors in Healthcare: A Concordat from the National Quality Board (2013) supported by the Chartered Institute of Ergonomics and Human Factors and other national bodies
- **https://www.researchgate.net/profile/Jeanette-Jackson/publication/266050169_Human_Factors_in_Patient_Safety_Review_of_Topics_and_Tools/**

links/55cb14d708aea2d9bdcc192e/Human-Factors-in-Patient-Safety-Review-of-Topics-and-Tools.pdf WHO (2009) Human Factors in Patient Safety: Review of Topics and Tools

Run charts:

* **https://www.ncbi.nlm.nih.gov/pmc/articles/PMC7337871/**

Part 2

Developing skills for quality improvement: Introducing Elisabeth

Catherine Delves-Yates and Gillian Janes

This second part of the textbook will enable you to understand how important it is to work with others to identify the need for improvement, make the changes required and to evaluate the result if quality improvement is to occur. We will be considering a range of different ways you can do this, and we will consider some of the challenges you may meet. In a similar way to Part 1 of the book, the material and activities in the following chapters will also help you to understand the terminology used and, most importantly, continue to recognise how quality improvement can become a feature of your everyday practice.

At the start of each chapter you will hear from some registered nurses and nursing students, who are very likely to be sharing the challenges and asking the questions you are, as you work upon developing your quality improvement skills.

Before you start to read the chapters in this part, however, we would like to introduce you to Elisabeth Chandler, who is going to share her thoughts about an idea where current practice could be improved. As you read what Elisabeth says, you will see how she has applied the ideas we explored in Part 1 such as adopting an 'improvement mind-set' during her placement experiences. As we progress through this part of the book we will refer to Elisabeth and identify how she could build on the improvement idea she has identified and develop the improvement skills she will need to take effective action to improve the situation.

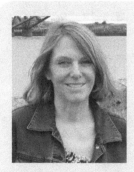 Hello! My name is Elisabeth Chandler. I am 32 and am a second-year nursing student, currently just about to finish my last placement this year. It has been a busy year so I am looking forward to my summer break! I started the nursing programme as a mature student; before I came into nursing I worked in journalism for several years. I am so pleased that I made the decision to change careers, and interestingly, the understanding of the importance of effective communication I gained from journalism has been really helpful in my nursing programme so far.

(Continued)

(Continued)

I have just finished a lecture where, to prepare for the final year of the nursing programme, it has been explained what we are going to be focusing upon for our theory assignment when we come back from summer break. I am really excited about this assignment, as I am going to be undertaking a quality improvement project, and I think I already have an excellent idea as to what I can focus upon.

So far in my nursing programme I have undertaken four placements in different care areas, both in the community and in hospitals. I have really enjoyed this experience, but if I reflect upon what I have seen, there is one area in all of my placement experiences where I feel there is a need for improvement.

We have been told in numerous lectures how important communication is. I remember one lecturer particularly telling us about the importance of communication in the delivery of effective patient-centred care. This was mainly focused upon the quality of communication between patients and clinicians, but there was discussion about how it is also known that poor communication is a major factor in healthcare errors, and that poor staff 'handover' of patient information is a problem. If we do not communicate effectively with other members of the team during 'handover', the potential result for patients is at best a poor experience of care and at worst a negative impact on both their safety and clinical outcomes.

In my placements so far, I have come to realise that giving an effective nursing handover is a difficult skill to master. I have worked with some nurses who were really good at it, but I have also received some handovers that were far from informative. I also had a very interesting placement where handover was given at the patient bedside, which was excellent in the way that patients were involved in the process, but I was concerned about confidentiality, as it was easy for other patients and visitors to hear what was being discussed.

In my previous experience as a journalist, when gathering material and making reports I used a range of 'aide memoires', which really were just hints and tips that helped me to remember what I needed to find out and then include in my report. In my placement experience I have been surprised that none of the areas had a specific tool for staff to use to ensure the handover they gave didn't miss out any important information and was as effective as possible. The nurses who I thought gave good handovers did share their information in a systematic way. Conversely, one of the biggest problems with the nurses who didn't give good handovers was that they didn't have any structure to what they were saying – they flipped backwards and forwards between different bits of information, so I used to get lost.

So, over my summer break I am going to start investigating to see what specific 'aide memoire' I can find for my nursing handover. If I can find one that would fit all of the placement areas I have been in so far, I think this would be really useful and improve the effectiveness of information exchange between nurses – and also be very helpful for nursing students!

I am also thinking that, if nurses get used to using a particular 'tool' to share information at handover, it could be useful in other situations. For example, my most recent placement was in an area where it is unusual for patients to be physically unwell. One of the patients, however, got very sick and had a cardiac arrest, so the emergency team were called. The person leading the emergency team asked the nurse caring for the patient to tell her the patient's history. The nurse gave the best overview he could, but in such a stressful situation I could see he found it difficult to do, and what he said wasn't easy to follow. I think if nurses were used to using a structured way to share information during their everyday handover, using it during emergency situations would also be much easier. Thinking about this even more, it would also be true if staff were working in areas they were unfamiliar with – for example if they had gone to help in another area because there was a staff shortage. Knowing you have a good 'tool' or a 'formula' you could apply when you needed to share patient information would be useful everywhere!

So, I am going to spend some time finding relevant literature and reading it over the summer break, so when I start back for year 3 I have a lot of information as to the tools nurses can use to ensure they give the best handover of information they can. Then I can focus upon how I turn this information into a quality improvement project!

Chapter 3 · Leading change and working with others

Nickey Rooke and Mark Morson

NMC Future Nurse: Standards of Proficiency for Registered Nurses

This chapter will address the following platforms and proficiencies:

Platform 1: Being an accountable professional

1.11 communicate effectively using a range of skills and strategies with colleagues and people at all stages of life and with a range of mental, physical, cognitive and behavioural health challenges.

Platform 5: Leading and managing care and working in teams

5.1 understand the principles of effective leadership, management, group and organisational dynamics and culture and apply these to team working and decision-making.

Platform 6: Improving safety and quality of care

6.4 demonstrate an understanding of the principles of improvement methodologies, participate in all stages of audit activity and identify appropriate quality improvement strategies.

6.9 work with people, their families, carers and colleagues to develop effective improvement strategies for quality and safety, sharing feedback and learning from positive outcomes and experiences, mistakes and adverse outcomes and experiences.

Chapter aims

After reading this chapter you should be able to:

- apply change theory and the principles of leading change within the context of your role;
- explain the principles and practice of partnership working and the role of interdependent practice in quality improvement;
- demonstrate an awareness of and select appropriately from a range of quality improvement tools and techniques to support collaborative quality improvement in practice;
- critically explore personal influencing skills with reference to a range of factors affecting the successful leadership of change.

I remember feeling nervous about presenting my quality improvement idea; looking out and seeing a room full of ward managers and matrons. It was daunting presenting to people with so much clinical knowledge and experience. I was wary about how they perceived me and my idea, but I maintained a strong belief in my idea and that it could significantly improve care.

(Tilly, 3rd year learning disability nursing student)

No one knows if the service delivered is meeting the needs, aspirations and desires of service users other than service users themselves, and those who care for them. No amount of number crunching can come near to knowing if what is being done to the patient is also being done with them unless they are involved in quality improvement.

(Jeremy, service user)

Introduction

Understanding the principles of quality improvement and your own contributions as outlined in Chapter 2 are important first steps towards instigating change in practice; the next step is to think about how you can work with others to lead change and enhance the quality of care experienced by service users, carers and families. Leading change and working with others are fundamental components of contemporary UK Government health policy (NHS, 2019) and are included in the professional codes of practice of health professionals. Learning to lead and manage change are just as important proficiencies as clinical patient-centred practices but can be harder to distinguish because they are such an intrinsic part of our day-to-day practice. Plus, as Tilly identifies at the start of the chapter, it can feel very scary to share your ideas, especially with people you feel have greater knowledge and experience than you.

This chapter outlines the principles underpinning the ability to lead and manage change, highlighting how they can be applied within your role. As a fundamental aspect of quality improvement, we will focus upon working in partnership with a range of other individuals, considering specifically, as Jeremy's comment highlights, the importance of including those who use healthcare services. We will also explore how you can decide which tools to select from the many available to support collaborative quality improvement in your practice and how to develop and apply personal influencing skills to successfully lead change.

Principles of leading change

The NHS 'Long Term Plan' (NHS, 2019) sets out five ambitions for improvement to ensure that the NHS remains 'fit for the future' by:

1. doing things differently;
2. preventing illness and tackling health inequalities;
3. backing the workforce;
4. making better use of data and digital technology;
5. getting the most out of taxpayers' investment in the NHS.

To meet these, it is important for health professionals and academics to nurture the future workforce; helping students recognise their role as change agents and leaders of change. Chapter 2 introduced leadership in terms of leading improvement; we will explore this in more depth here, starting with the principles of leading change.

Activity 3.1   Reflection

Watch this four-minute video from the NHS Leadership Academy, where several pre-registration students discuss their understanding of leadership and how developing leadership skills will enable them to effect change to improve patient care:

https://www.youtube.com/watch?v=Sp8KfM4MQB8&t=17s

- List the leadership skills the students felt were necessary to become a good leader in practice.
- Think about the skills you need to develop or strengthen to lead change. During your next placement, discuss these with your practice assessor and identify some specific learning opportunities to help you achieve these learning objectives.

Good leadership skills are essential for successful change, but what makes a good change leader? Miller (2001) offers a three-point framework for change leadership that helps to answer this question. Change leadership is about our ability to recognise our personal capacity to adapt to change where we have learned to cope with situations or events that initially appear daunting or threatening. Leading change can be stressful, and leaders are often judged on their ability to remain calm despite the surrounding chaos. The second element is our internalised change beliefs. Miller (2001) argues that lessons learned from previous mistakes enable change leaders to shift their beliefs from supposing that everyone will change once they understand the need for flexibility, enabling them to use different improvement tools, leadership styles and behaviours, depending on the situation. Miller's (2001) final point refers to a change leader's behaviour and what they consciously or unconsciously do during the change process. Good leaders maintain focus; take time to ensure that the need and rationale for change is understood and that there is a shared vision and purpose; actively lead the change throughout from planning through implementation and evaluation; recognise the importance of networking; and are committed to adopting a systematic approach.

As has been clearly recognised in the Leading Change, Adding Value initiative (NHS England, 2016), good healthcare leaders specifically have a hugely important role in shaping the future while also managing current challenges. Many of these leadership skills align with the six Cs of nursing (DH, 2012); however, there are additional values and behaviours that you will need to incorporate into your practice specifically when leading a quality improvement project that involves change, as outlined in the eleven Cs for leading change in Table 3.1.

Eleven Cs for leading change	
Clarity	Ability to clearly communicate the need for change, project goals and objectives. Change leaders should provide accurate information using language that is easy to understand and avoids the use of professional jargon.
Critical thinking	Ability to look beyond what you initially see or hear, to explore the evidence base to validate assumptions or find better solutions.
Culture	Leaders must understand the culture of the team and organisation. Culture encompasses cultural awareness, cultural competence, cultural intelligence and cultural humility.
Collaboration	Required to foster open and inclusive relationships with key stakeholders, including service users, carers and families.
Communication	Leaders must communicate the purpose of change, what needs to change and why change is necessary. Requires the ability to listen to others, share ideas, build rapport and trust.
Courage	Leading change often requires a degree of courage; to problem-solve, manage disputes or conflict, to accept blame if things go wrong, but also to let go and trust others to complete their assigned tasks, roles and responsibilities.
Commitment	Leaders should be committed to the change, role-modelling the right values and behaviours, leading by example and inspiring those around them.
Compassion	Ability to be supportive and demonstrate empathy to the team, key stakeholders, colleagues and communities involved or affected by the change.
Confidence	Confidence grows through experience and believing in your ability to lead. This relates to having a sense of proportion, an ability to give praise and accept responsibility when things go wrong, and maintain a sense of humour.

Eleven Cs for leading change	
Creativity	Ability to look at problems from different perspectives and identify innovative solutions.
Credibility	Demonstrating the knowledge, skills and experience required to lead change. Requires honesty, openness and transparency.

Table 3.1   The eleven Cs for leading change

Applying change theory to practice

When instigating change we apply change theory to increase the chances of success. Essentially, we use change theory to help us achieve the desired result but, importantly, we use it before this, to work out exactly what the desired result is. As Mager (1997, pvi) outlines,

> *If you don't know where you're going, the best made maps won't help you get there.*

So, although change theory is often likened to a map enabling us to move to a new position, it is much more than this, and is used to underpin all the thinking and actions we undertake.

Supporting change from endings to new beginnings

Change is an inevitable part of life and within healthcare staff experience a perpetual cycle of organisational change at all levels. It is therefore important to consider the psychological impact change can have on colleagues, people accessing services and their families. When we consider change, we think about it in terms of moving from one state to another. Lewin's change management model illustrates this, as shown in Figure 3.1.

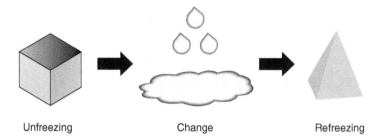

| Unfreezing | Change | Refreezing |

Figure 3.1   Lewin's Change Management Theory (1951)

The change process is often represented as an ice cube that changes its state by melting and refreezing into another state.

Applying this to a change in practice, to 'unfreeze' you must clearly identify what needs changing. This may require you look at data, including for example service user feedback, staff surveys and audit results, to understand the current situation. Analysing data and talking to colleagues and service users enables you to establish a clearer picture of the charge required, understand why change is necessary and determine how to communicate the need for change to others. This is also the time to establish who the key stakeholders are by conducting a stakeholder analysis, as first introduced in Chapters 1 and 2. During the 'change' stage, represented in Figure 3.1 by a 'puddle', individuals start to transition from their current position towards a new desired state. In the 'change' stage, we can assess the balance between the forces that are driving the change and those resisting it, as shown in Figure 3.2.

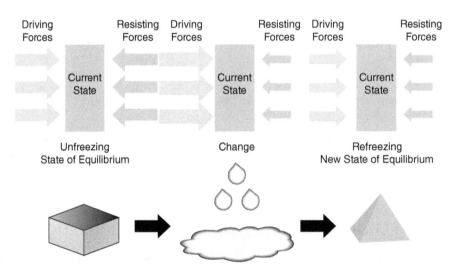

Figure 3.2   Lewin's Force Field Analysis (Lewin, 1951)

Figure 3.2 shows how, during 'unfreezing', equilibrium is initially maintained as the driving forces are in balance with the resisting forces; change can only occur when the driving forces are stronger than those in opposition, which prevents the current state being maintained. Eventually, if people have accepted new ways of working and established new practices and behaviours (refreezing), the desired state of change is achieved. The application of these ideas is illustrated further in Chapter 5.

Becoming a change agent: understanding individuals' transition to change

To support people through change, it is important to appreciate the psychological impact change can have on them. William Bridges identified three transitional stages that we experience when encountering change. Bridges (1991) argues that change and transition are two distinct **concepts**; while change is usually centred on a particular event or situation, transition is associated with the psychological processes we go through as we begin to adapt and change our own values, emotions and behaviours in response (Leybourne, 2016). Figure 3.3 illustrates how change often elicits a sense of discomfort as we move away from what we consider 'normal' practice – our comfort zone – into unchartered territory where we may experience intense negative emotions as our established ways of working become challenged. The 'Transition' phase is described as the 'neutral zone', where we move from 'what was' to 'what will be' (Bridges, 1991, p44). While this can still create negative emotions such as apathy, resentment and resistance, as we move through the neutral zone we begin to learn new knowledge and skills, subsequently becoming more motivated and increasingly confident because we begin to understand why change is necessary. In the final phase, 'New Beginnings', we move into the growth zone where we start to embrace and accept change, become familiar with new practices or ways of thinking, recognising the learning that has taken place and showing a renewed commitment to our role and the wider team.

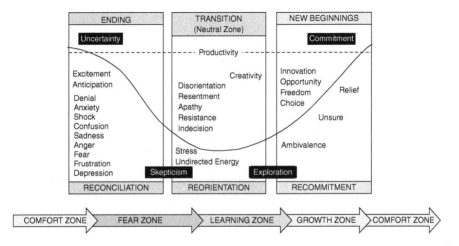

Figure 3.3 Bridge's Transition Model (1991) and associated zones of comfort

You may wish to explore other transition models, such as the Kubler-Ross change curve (EKR Foundation, 2022), which is based on her 'Five Stages of Grief', or Fisher's Transition Curve (2012) that combine aspects of the Kubler-Ross and Bridges models. It is important to recognise that although these models are not change management tools, they do provide valuable insight into how change can affect those around you.

Activity 3.2 Critical thinking

Click on this link to watch Darin Rowell outlining ways in which a leader can understand and manage the transition phase: https://www.youtube.com/watch?v=jhConwpzjQ0

Next, consider Elisabeth's improvement project and answer these questions:

(Continued)

(Continued)

- Who are the people who will be affected by the change Elisabeth proposes?
- List some of the possible different expectations people might have about her idea.
- What different types of resistance or losses may emerge?
- How could Elisabeth mitigate against or manage resistance?

Compare your responses with those in the relevant activities answer at the end of this chapter.

For any quality improvement project to be successful, it is vital individuals are supported through the transitional period. Figure 3.4 outlines several useful strategies that can be used to do so.

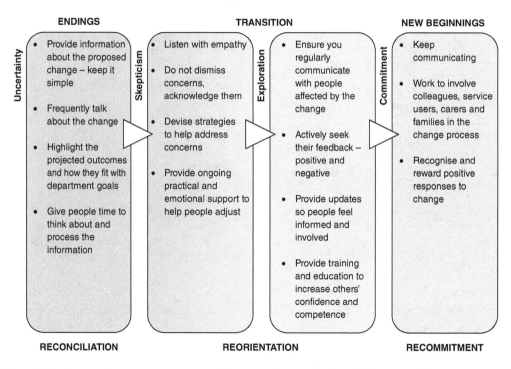

Figure 3.4 Strategies to support transition to change (adapted from Rooke and Phipps, 2022)

Activity 3.3   Building knowledge

Using your online information searching skills, find the NHS Change Model Guide (2018) (NHS England), and read the information provided.

Keep this information in mind as you read through the rest of this section of the chapter.

The NHS Change Model

The NHS Change Model Guide (NHS England, 2018) supports the use of the eight-part NHS Change Model, a framework originally developed in 2012 with health professionals to support change, large or small.

This model goes some way to address the criticism that linear frameworks such as Lewin (1951) and Bridges (1991) promote an overly simplistic step-by-step approach to change, and concern that they do not adequately reflect the complexities of public sector organisations. Instead, the NHS Change Model Guide (2018) offers an integrated framework, in which each of the eight components can be revisited throughout the change cycle, although all have equal value and remain interdependent (Martin et al, 2013).

The interdependence of the eight components becomes more apparent when we consider some of the key questions associated with each (see Table 3.2), which can be used to support any quality improvement.

NHS Change Model components	Some key questions to consider
	(taken from The Change Model 'Key Questions', NHS Improving Quality, 2014; NHS England, 2018)
Shared purpose	How do I create a co-produced shared purpose?
	What will I do to show that everyone has equal value in the planning, design, delivery and evaluation?
	How does everyone benefit from the change?
	Does this improvement meet that shared purpose?
Spread and adoption	How are we going to spread good practice and innovation?
Improvement tools	Are we using correct evidence-based improvement tools for our change and how can patients influence this?
	How can we enable patients to challenge our improvement method?
	How are patients' experiences reflected in our approach to change?
Project and performance management	What is our roadmap for improvement and change and how will we know how far down the road we are?
	How are we going to review progress and realign if necessary?
	How will we know if the milestones remain right as the change progresses?
	How do we ensure all stakeholders continue to buy into the change?
Transparent measurement	Are we measuring the planned or actual impact of change correctly?
	How can staff and patients help us understand the whole picture and create shared ownership?
	How can we ensure our plans are transparent?
	What milestones will be identified so that we remain on track to achieve our shared purpose?

(Continued)

Table 3.2   (Continued)

System drivers	What processes, incentives and systems are in place to support change?
	What is the problem we are trying to fix?
	What are the real reasons for change?
Motivate and mobilise	Are we engaging and mobilising all the right people?
	How will I motivate and mobilise people?
	What is the patient's role and how will we support them, so their voice is heard?
	How can I show that engagement strategies were successful?
Leadership by all	Do we have the leadership skills to create transformational change?
	How are we enabling shared leadership?
	How are we able to demonstrate that patients and their families are influencing decisions?
	How do we communicate the need for change in a way that creates trust?
	How will people tell the difference they have made to the change and the influence they have had?

Table 3.2   NHS Change Model key questions

The NHS Change Model Guide (2018) offers a useful framework that can be applied to support the implementation of any quality improvement seeking to achieve transformational and sustainable change. Supporting individuals and encouraging them to be part of change begins at the very start of any quality improvement, so a skill to develop is the ability to communicate your ideas for change in a way that not only clearly outlines their benefit, but also inspires others to want to become involved.

Communicating ideas and leading change

Earlier in this chapter we considered how leaders can effectively communicate the purpose of change, what needs to be changed, and why change is necessary. To help you outline your change ideas effectively, an 'APIE approach', focusing upon issues of **A**ssessment, **P**lanning, **I**mplementation, and **E**valuation (APIE) can be useful. APIE forms part of the nursing process (Orlando, 1961) and is frequently used in nursing practice. In a similar way to using the APIE approach to provide care, the stages can be used to guide the effective communication of quality improvement ideas. Table 3.3 outlines how Elisabeth could use this approach when communicating her handover tool idea to stakeholders.

Assessment	• How are you going to communicate your idea?
	• What is your aim(s)?

An important initial assessment is to consider the aims of the communication. There may be varying aims depending on the context of the discussion. For example, Elisabeth might be pitching her idea for the first time to an audience of clinical leaders, so an aim could be to gain their support. Alternatively, she might be explaining to staff how to use the handover tool, so the aim would be to educate and develop understanding.

It is always important to ensure that you have considered the stakeholder position, so Elisabeth needs to ask herself how her audience might affect or be affected by the change, taking into account the audience's prior knowledge and experiences in relation to the change.

Elisabeth should also assess the time and resources available, as well as the environment the discussion will take place in, as these will inform the planning stage.

Planning	• How best can I achieve my aim or aims?
	• What will inspire others to want to become involved?

A good starting point for the planning stage is to carefully consider the time available to communicate an idea. Relating this to Elisabeth and her audience, they may have a protected window of time to discuss the idea at length. Elisabeth should capitalise on this and plan for a comprehensive discussion about her idea. Alternatively, the time available may be limited, so it could be necessary to prepare a more concise discussion. If time is very short, Elisabeth could consider engaging with her audience through a different medium; by email, leaflets or a poster for example.

If directly engaging her audience, the environment will influence how Elisabeth plans to discuss her idea. She may be required to discuss her idea in settings such as a boardroom, a staff room or a hospital cafeteria, so will need to consider factors such as privacy, risk of interruption, noise levels and how these might impact discussion. For example, a formal presentation might be practical in a boardroom, but impractical in a busy cafeteria, so an informal discussion would be better. Elisabeth could also explore discussing her idea remotely through a virtual meeting if she is unable to find a suitable venue.

It is also helpful to consider the IT resources available when planning a discussion. Technological resources can be particularly helpful, and will enable Elisabeth to communicate in inventive ways, by designing an imaginative and engaging presentation. For example, if Elisabeth can access film editing software, she could record her presentation and eliminate the need to present her idea in person altogether.

The careful planning of the content of the discussion is also important. In order to gain support from others, Elisabeth needs her content to be inspiring and able to captivate her audience's imagination. She will also need to include a clear rationale outlining the benefits of implementing the change, with an up-to-date, relevant evidence base to support this. When planning to communicate an idea it is always important to plan content which the audience will find relevant and engaging, and deliver it at a level that is easy to follow.

(Continued)

Table 3.3 (Continued)

Implementation	• Communicate the change with passion and confidence

When communicating with her audience directly, it is particularly important that Elisabeth clearly explains her idea. It is understandable that she may feel nervous, which can negatively impact on presenting behaviours. According to Van Emden and Becker (2016), skilled speakers use a combination of effective verbal and non-verbal communication, varying the volume, pitch, and tempo of their speech to emphasise key points. They also use effective non-verbal communication, making eye contact and maintaining an open body posture to maximise engagement with the audience. These are strategies Elisabeth can also apply.

Evaluation	• What was good?
	• What can be better?

Evaluation enables reflection on actions to improve subsequent practice. Gaining feedback directly from the audience, who are very likely to offer useful and helpful insights, is a good way for Elisabeth to do this. Even if the communication was indirect (such as emails, leaflets or posters) it is possible to gain feedback by reviewing responses and uptake. The feedback gained can then be implemented in order to ensure future communication is as effective as possible.

Table 3.3 Using an APIE approach to communicate a change idea

Leading change and influencing others

In the previous section we discussed how Elisabeth might approach communicating her idea, with a key aim of gaining support from others. Accordingly, when implementing a quality improvement, being able to persuade and influence others is a very useful skill. While this may sound daunting, there are techniques you can apply to help, and like any skill, the more you practice the better you will become.

A good starting point is offered by Cialdini (2009), who describes six principles by which individuals are persuaded, and Table 3.4 outlines how to apply these principles when communicating your idea to others.

Principle	Description
Reciprocity	Individuals are more persuaded by those they are indebted to, feeling compelled to exchange or repay a previous favour.
Commitment and consistency	The practice of standing by (in word and deed) a previous statement or action is highly valued in all cultures.
Social proof	We look to those around us to determine what to believe or how to act in a situation.
Liking	Simply put, people are much more likely to say yes to those they know and like.
Authority	We are likely to comply with the request of someone we see as an authority.
Scarcity	The scarcer the commodity, the more people want it, as we assign more value to the things that are less available.

Table 3.4 Cialdini's six principles of persuasion (adapted from Clark and Kemp, 2008)

The principles highlighted in Table 3.4 outline some points to consider when leading change and sharing our ideas with others. It is fundamentally important, however, that we are always ethical in our use of persuasion and influencing. The relationship between persuasion, influencing, deception, coercion and manipulation is complex, but there are two values that must always be upheld:

1. Leaders must never knowingly deceive or manipulate others and never distort or knowingly omit certain truths.

2. Individuals must not be made to feel coerced into supporting an idea; autonomy to offer or withhold support must always be respected.

Principles of interdependent working

Chapter 1 asked you to think about stakeholders and complete a stakeholder analysis of Harry's stakeholders. Building on this, we now introduce the concept of interdependent working, to help you consider how to work more effectively with key stakeholders to lead change. In your previous stakeholder analysis, you considered the levels of involvement and commitment required from each of Harry's stakeholders. The next step is to establish the degree of dependence, independence and interdependency the stakeholders have with each other; this is especially important at the beginning of any quality improvement.

Defining interdependence

In healthcare, we often talk about interdependent, multidisciplinary or interprofessional working. This involves us each playing our part within the wider healthcare system, collaborating with other professional groups, service users, families and carers to achieve the best outcomes for each person. We must therefore consider what is meant by the terms dependence, independence and interdependence in view of working with others to lead a quality improvement, as identified in Table 3.5.

Dependence	• Project team members depend on the leader to make key decisions and start each phase of the project.
	• Team members are dependent on the leader for direction, recognition and approval.
Independence	• The project team are encouraged to use their own initiative and intrinsic desire to achieve the quality improvement objectives.
	• Independent team members are empowered to develop personal and professional autonomy and **self-efficacy**.
	• Each team member can work on different parts of the quality improvement, bringing it back to the group for discussion and approval.

(Continued)

Table 3.5 (Continued)

Interdependence	• Each member of the team has a shared vision and common goals that are mutually beneficial.
	• Team members subsequently develop balanced, reciprocal relationships that promote collaborative working.
	• All recognise the value of each other's contributions and how that positively impacts on the outcomes.

Table 3.5 A comparison of dependence, independence and interdependence in quality improvement

Bases of interconnectedness

Table 3.5 showed that interdependence consists of what Sebok-Syer et al (2021, p2) describe as 'patterns of interactions between individuals that influence experience and outcomes'. In quality improvement, while each member of the team may work independently at times, everyone's roles and responsibilities are interconnected, much like cogs in a machine. As such, we are interdependent on each other to ensure that the quality improvement objectives are achieved, often referred to as '*outcome interdependence*' (Wageman, 1995). Such interdependence is underpinned by four bases of interconnectedness that link members of any team together, as shown in Figure 3.5.

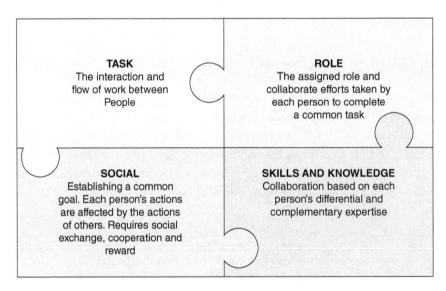

Figure 3.5 A conceptual framework of interdependence (Penning, 1975)

As a leader of change, it is important to consider each of these four bases and the leadership style needed to enable key stakeholders to work together productively. While each base is important, Penning (1975) argues that interdependence is grounded at the task level where the tasks or actions each person carries out are related to and have consequences for the completion of ongoing and future actions.

This might appear to suggest that one task must be completed before the next person can start the next task; this is referred to as *sequential interdependence*. However, as illustrated in Figure 3.6, tasks might have *reciprocal interdependence* where people or teams work independently on different tasks, while also exchanging or working on tasks between themselves. Where there is no independency between tasks, the notion of *pooled interdependence* applies, where everyone's individual efforts collectively contribute to the overall success of the project. Finally, *intensive interdependence* relies on strong communication links, problem solving and simultaneous and collective collaboration (Thompson, 1967).

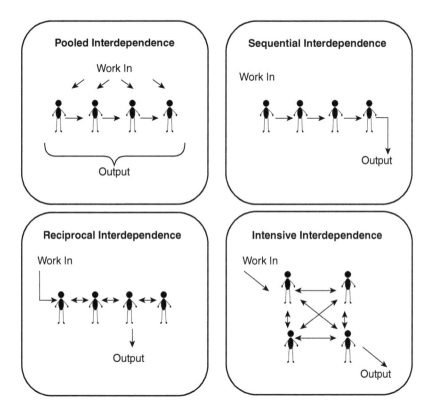

Figure 3.6 Types of task interdependence (adapted from Mach et al, 2021)

Activity 3.4   Team working

Interdependency mapping

Building on Activity 1.3 in Chapter 1 where you identified Harry's stakeholders, the purpose of this activity is for you to explore and appreciate the social interactions and interconnectedness between individuals and groups, and how these interconnections could be applied when introducing a quality improvement initiative in practice.

(Continued)

(*Continued*)

Look at the Part 2 Introduction to Elisabeth and her quality improvement idea regarding 'aide memoires' to improve nursing handovers. Create an interconnectedness or social network map that identifies all the people or teams Elisabeth will need to work with to achieve her aim and the levels of interdependence between them by following these instructions:

- Take a piece of A4 paper and place Elisabeth at the centre of the page, drawing a circle around her.
- On a separate piece of paper or small Post-It notes list all the people, teams or groups that Elisabeth will need to work with, talk to or involve in her project.
- Place all the people, teams or groups that Elisabeth will most frequently need to work with close to her on the A4 mapping document, and place those who Elisabeth will work with less frequently further away from her.

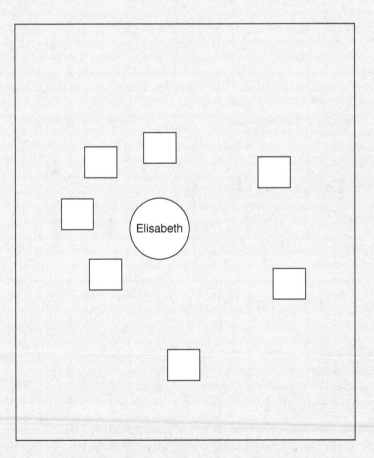

- What you have drawn can be referred to as a 'mapping document'. Review the mapping document and if you think there are people, teams or groups that will regularly interact or work together, move them closer together.

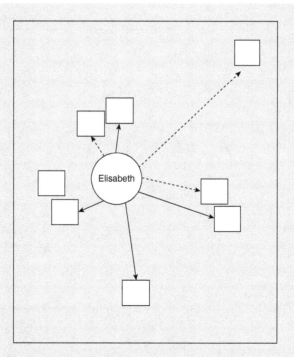

- Using a blue pen, draw an arrow from Elisabeth to any of the people, teams or groups that she will need to regularly communicate with about the project. Use a dotted blue line for any weak communication connections.

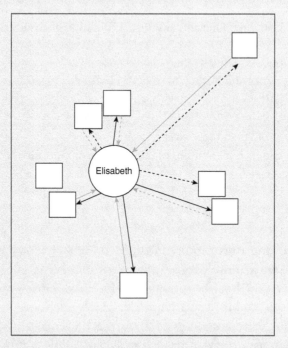

- Next, use a red pen to draw arrows from the people, teams or groups who will regularly communicate with or provide information to Elisabeth, again use a dotted red line for any weak communication connections.

(Continued)

(Continued)

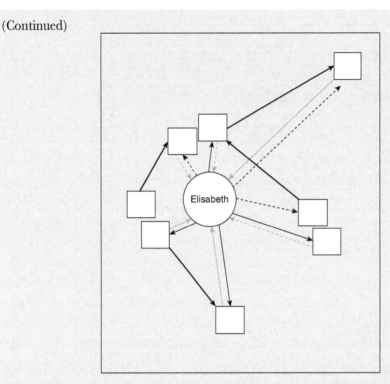

- Finally, use a green pen to draw arrows between different people, teams or groups who will communicate and share information with each other.

Review your interdependency map and answer the following questions:

- Who does Elisabeth have the strongest connections with?
- How much influence might they have over Elisabeth's project (are they supportive, neutral or restrictive)?
- Who does Elisabeth have the weakest connections with?
- How could she strengthen those connections?
- How will these connections and interdependencies support Elisabeth in implementing her quality improvement idea?

Interdependent working thus requires leaders to actively engage with stakeholders so they can collectively achieve project objectives that bring about positive improvements in healthcare and health outcomes. This links closely with the concept of collective leadership introduced in Chapter 2, which encourages integrative and collaborative working for the common good. This is achieved by delegating leadership to those within the team with relevant expertise, skills and motivation (West et al, 2014). Collective leadership can result in each person within the team understanding their role, using their skills and expertise to advance the quality improvement project, taking responsibility for their assigned tasks and developing collegiate social networks that foster productive, interdependent working practices.

Involving service users, carers and families in leading change

Involving service users, carers and families in leading change is a fundamental element of any quality improvement project. Service user involvement is embedded in UK health policy, which calls for all healthcare organisations to actively engage in collaborative co-production with service users, carers and their families. To achieve this it is important to consider what we mean by 'co-production' and 'service user involvement', and how these two terms are interrelated. Activity 3.5 encourages you to explore your current mind-set regarding service user, carer and family involvement.

Activity 3.5   Reflection

Reflect on your experiences of involving people, their carers or families in decisions about their care.

- How actively involved was the person, their carer or family in the decision-making process?
- Who decided what the treatment or care goals were – was it the service user, the health professional or was it a collaborative decision?
- If it was a collaborative decision, what did the health professional do to ensure that the service user, carer or family were involved as equal and active partners?

As this activity is based on your own reflection, there is no template answer at the end of the chapter; however, you may wish to discuss your notes/thoughts with your practice assessor or lecturer.

It doesn't serve the patient, the NHS, or the healthcare professionals well if therapy follows ritualistically along textbook lines without asking, 'is this actually working?'. Patients and the public should be involved in the design of services from the outset. For example, what is the point in holding a clinic always at the same time on the same day if the patient's work means they can't get to the clinic, or if the car park is too busy at that time of day, or if shifts end at the same time as school pick-up time so roads and traffic are heavy? We all have our little bubbles, unable to see beyond them, but involving patients and the public who live outside those bubbles can bring a unique perspective and should be an asset.

(Jeremy, Service User)

The questions in Activity 3.5 helped illustrated the extent to which service users, carers and their families are involved in making decisions about their care. Their involvement in quality improvement may initially seem fairly abstract, yet as Jeremy highlights, we must remember that service users, carers and families are the actual users of health services, and therefore should be involved not only in decisions about their care but also those concerning broader service delivery so that we fully appreciate their experiences, listen to their ideas for change and enable them to help lead the improvement process.

As introduced in Chapter 2, co-production is the way in which we work in equal partnership with people who use health and social care services; including involving them in designing, developing and evaluating services. Co-production recognises that a person's lived experience enables them to share their perspective on what it is like to be a recipient of health services. In turn, this helps health professionals and healthcare providers to ensure that services are person- and family-centred and reflect the reality of that lived experience. Therefore, to co-produce a quality improvement, we should actively involve service users, carers and families, moving away from tokenistic approaches such as providing information about a proposed improvement or engaging in consultation activities that often have little impact on the change made. When leading change, we must recognise the legitimacy of the person's experience and acknowledge that people who use health services should be enabled to act as 'critical friends' (Rowland et al, 2018).

There are ten key principles (see Table 3.6) for involving people in quality improvement that you can use to guide your own improvement activities to ensure the experiences of those who use services help shape and lead change.

Representativeness	Needs to reflect the diversity of the local population.
	Use targeted invitations.
Inclusivity	Removal of barriers that prevent active involvement: levels of health literacy, reasonable adjustments, accessibility (physical, cognitive, sensory), power imbalances, lack of knowledge of organisational structure or hierarchies.
Equality	To be treated equally and valued for their contributions, skills, knowledge and experience.
Sensitivity	To be sensitive about how meetings are conducted, the language, tone and actions taken.
Commitment	Committed to shared principles and values. Committed to listening and changing in response to service user, carer and family feedback.
Cultural sensitivity	To be sensitive and responsive to cultural differences including people's expectations, preferences, communication and use of language.
Transparency	To communicate honestly, clearly and openly.
	Ensure that the roles and responsibilities for people are clear and that everyone understands what they will contribute and how they will work with other members of the team.
Timeliness	To be involved from the beginning and consistently throughout the project. Avoid one-off, infrequent events.
Feedback	To be provided with regular feedback on how their contributions have influenced the direction of the quality improvement.
	Service users to be in control of the project's information dissemination process.
Remuneration	To provide remuneration for travel, time spent reading project documents, attending meetings etc.

Table 3.6 Ten fundamental principles for effective service user, carer and family involvement (adapted from National Survivor User Network, 2015 and HQIP, 2017)

Activity 3.6 provides an opportunity for you to apply these principles in a practice context.

Activity 3.6 Critical thinking

Go back to Chapter 2, Activity 2.6 and the example of Sia, who acted on a child's feedback that they were frightened by 'shadow monsters' at night. Sia had already highlighted some potential areas for improvement including repositioning lights and quiet closing waste bins. The senior nurse forum was supportive and asked her to put her ideas in action. Sia wanted to actively involve children, carers and families to help her make those proposals a reality; however, despite them knowing about the proposed changes, no one had expressed an interest in getting involved.

Using the ten principles for effective involvement, answer the following questions:

- List three strategies that Sia could adopt to encourage patients, carers and families to be involved in helping her solve this problem.
- What could Sia do to ensure that the children's, carers' and families' voices are heard?
- What can Sia do to support patients, carers and families to understand the whole picture and create a shared ownership for the change needed?
- How could Sia demonstrate where patients, carers and their families have influenced decisions about the change?

Note down your thoughts and then compare them with the example answer at the end of this chapter.

Leading change and challenging established workplace cultures

In Chapter 2, we met Brian, who experienced resistance when trying to introduce improvement that changed the existing way of working. When Brian reflects upon this, it is important that he recognises resistance to change can serve positive purposes. An organisation that blindly implements every new idea is equally as problematic as one that resists change (Hewitt-Taylor, 2013). What is important is to understand types of resistance. In Brian's experience, he found 'when I wasn't there, they just did what they had always done'. Parkin (2009) describes this as passive resistance, whereby individuals do not openly state their opposition to change; they may even express support, but their actions are contradictory. Other individuals may actively resist change and openly challenge new ways of practice. A degree of criticality to new ideas is beneficial, as this information can ensure all the implications for services and practice that a change may bring are rigorously considered before implementation.

For Brian to develop this change further, he needs to understand the issues underpinning the types of resistance facing him and use this to inform how he proceeds. A key factor of resistance can be that individuals may not understand the potential benefits of the proposed change. This may translate into active or passive resistance, or even result in apathy. Table 3.7 summarises various approaches to implementing change.

Approach	Description
Power–coercive	Power and fear of consequence of not engaging is used to drive change
Empirical–rational	If people understand why the change is needed and can see the benefits of it, they will participate.
Normative–reductive	Social and cultural implications of change are important factors determining why people accept or reject innovation.

Table 3.7 Approaches to change management (Chin and Benne, 1985)

The approaches to change identified in Table 3.7 can be associated with inherent problems. For example, using a power–coercive approach is not collaborative and therefore likely to generate resistance. To make change more acceptable, it is always wise to apply an empirical–rational approach, so there is an understanding of the need for change, and from a normative–reductive perspective, to ensure the proposed change is both socially and culturally appropriate.

Conclusion

All quality improvement involves change of some degree or another; therefore learning to lead and manage change are important skills to develop and practice in preparation for becoming a registered professional. This chapter has sought to strengthen your understanding of the psychological impact of change and the transitional processes people go through to be able to accept change, while identifying effective strategies you can apply to support this.

We have highlighted how change models and frameworks can be helpful in guiding you through the change process, from devising a shared purpose to identifying strategies for partnership and interdependent working, involving people accessing services and challenging established workplace cultures. You will need to draw on these broad principles and approaches as you move on to consider how to identify and justify an improvement idea in the next chapter.

Glossary

Concepts: abstract ideas or notions
Self-efficacy: an individual's belief in their capacity to act in the ways necessary to reach specific goals

Answers to activities

Activity 3.1 Reflection

Leadership skills students felt were necessary to become a good leader in practice:

- understanding teams/systems/care delivery;
- confidence;
- inclusivity;
- reflection;
- self-leadership;
- delegation;
- communication;
- multidimensional aspect of leadership;
- self-belief;
- self-care;
- open mind;
- honesty.

Activity 3.2 Critical thinking

There are numerous answers for this activity; this is not an exhaustive list – you may well have thought of many that we have not included!

Who are the people that are going to be affected by the change Elisabeth is proposing?

- nurses, other healthcare professionals, patients, carers.

List some of the possible differences in expectation people might have about her idea.

They may or may not think it will:

- be difficult to achieve;
- take lots of time;
- take lots of effort;
- work;
- be a good idea;
- achieve an improvement.

What are the different types of resistance or losses that may emerge?

- loss of choice of handover format;
- resistance due to lack of understanding, not wanting to follow the identified format, apathy.

How could Elisabeth mitigate or manage resistance?

- involve others in the change to gain their support;
- seek out the views of people who are unsupportive of the change, listen to and address their concerns;
- constantly seek feedback and address any negative issues;
- communicate effectively with all involved.

Activity 3.4 Team working

Who does Elisabeth have the strongest connections with?

- Nursing staff (both registered and non-registered).

How much influence might they have over Elisabeth's project (are they supportive, neutral or restrictive)?

- The nursing staff may be all of these – supportive, neutral or restrictive depending upon their view of the change. This clearly demonstrates how important it is to enable the nursing staff involved in the change to fully understand the importance of what is being implemented and that they are involved in it, to ensure they can highlight their views and feel listened to.

Who does Elisabeth have the weakest connections with?

- Non-nursing healthcare professionals.

How could she strengthen those connections?

- Ensure they have information about the change and offer them the opportunity to be involved in its planning and implementation.

How will these connections and interdependencies support Elisabeth in implementing her quality improvement idea?

- Involving other healthcare professionals will enable Elisabeth to receive further feedback and advice upon the change and gain support for what is being implemented. This will not only be practically useful but will also be motivating.

Activity 3.6 Critical thinking

List three strategies Sia could adopt to encourage patients, carers and families to help her solve this problem?

- Ask them for their ideas.
- Have a display board explaining the improvement and invite them to add their ideas.
- Ask the play therapist for assistance to get the children's views.

What could Sia do to ensure that the children's, carers' and families' voices are heard?

- Integrate them in her plan for change.
- Share them with colleagues in the organisation.

What can Sia do to support the children, carers and families in understanding the whole picture and create shared ownership for the change needed?

- Involve them as members of the team introducing change.

How could Sia demonstrate where patients, carers and their families have influenced decisions about the change?

- Capture their thoughts and identify the specific areas where their views have been integrated in the plan.

Chapter 4   Identifying and justifying the need for service improvement

Gillian Janes and Catherine Delves-Yates

NMC Future Nurse: Standards of Proficiency for Registered Nurses

This chapter will address the following platforms and proficiencies:

Platform 1: Being an accountable professional

1.8 demonstrate the knowledge, skills and ability to think critically when applying evidence and drawing on experience to make informed decisions in all situations.

Platform 6: Improving safety and quality of care

6.4 demonstrate an understanding of the principles of improvement methodologies, participate in all stages of audit activity and identify appropriate quality improvement strategies.

6.7 understand how the quality and effectiveness of nursing care can be evaluated in practice, and demonstrate how to use service delivery evaluation and audit findings to bring about continuous improvement.

Platform 7: Co-ordinating care

7.12 demonstrate understanding of the processes involved in developing a basic business case for additional care funding by applying knowledge of finance, resources and safe staffing levels.

Chapter aims

After reading this chapter you should be able to:

- demonstrate an awareness of a range of appropriate evidence that can be used to identify quality improvements in practice;
- determine appropriate quality improvement-based solutions in practice based on evaluation of potential options, using relevant tools and frameworks;
- understand how to scope a sustainable quality improvement idea;
- understand the importance of planning to evaluate and measure the effectiveness of the improvement project.

It seemed obvious to me from my first day that people got bored and more anxious the longer they had to wait to be seen. They were probably worried about the consultation and had nothing else to think about except watching the clock. Why aren't we capitalising upon this 'free time' by making a range of health promotion leaflets available in the waiting area?

(Shella, student nurse, GP surgery)

Introduction

Previous chapters have explored the nurse's role in improvement, and enabled you to assess and develop your improvement capability and how to work effectively with others to lead change. However, before any change can be implemented, a specific improvement intervention must first be identified and then justified, not only to convince others to support it, as successful, sustainable change is collaborative, but also to ensure there is benefit for all involved.

Identifying the need for improvement and then the appropriate solution is not always straightforward. Often, especially when you are new to an area of practice or context, ideas for improvement may jump out at you; this may be excellent practice you have seen elsewhere (sometimes termed 'learning from excellence' or 'positive deviance') or ways to enhance current care processes or outcomes (as we saw with Harry in Part 1 of this book). Such revelations can be a consequence of the 'fresh eyes' perspective we discussed in Chapter 1, or perhaps you bring a particularly curious or creative attitude to your work. However, what seems obvious to you may not even be recognised or viewed with the same motivation for change by colleagues. You may already have found yourself in this position, in a similar way to Shella, who shared her thoughts with us at the start of the chapter. While Shella's idea may be a good one, she needs to explore potential solutions and investigate the evidence to determine what the best solution might be. Ensuring there is evidence to underpin any improvement is crucial, plus as we learned in Chapter 3, influencing and persuading others is an important improvement skill that often also involves justifying any proposed change.

When undertaking a small or student-led improvement as part of a learning programme, for example, it is very unlikely you will be required to submit a formal **business case**, though more information on this is provided in the further reading section at the end of the chapter if needed. What you will need to do, however, is address all the issues that a formal business case would require you to consider. This involves providing a sound, evidence-based rationale for any proposed change, generating and appraising potential solutions to arrive at a well-justified recommendation for change or intervention that considers a wide range of relevant factors. As with a formal business case, this will need to include a cost–benefit analysis, therefore increasing your knowledge of how and when to draw on the specialist knowledge of colleagues, e.g. business development manager is a key element of developing your improvement skills. This type of comprehensive background analysis and justification is an effective means of ensuring precious time and other resources are targeted appropriately, but also crucially, of convincing others to lend their support or, if necessary, give permission for you to proceed (Carter, 2017). This chapter will therefore focus on the sources and types of evidence that can be used to identify and justify improvement, how to generate and appraise potential solutions and effectively **scope** a sustainable response based on effective, collaborative planning for evaluation and measurement.

Evidence informed improvement

Any aspect of nursing practice should be evidence informed and, regardless of whether an improvement effort aims to enhance or spread excellent practice or address a problem or challenge, data is key. As this definition illustrates:

> *Quality improvement (QI) describes systematic, data-guided activities designed to bring about immediate, positive changes in the delivery of healthcare in particular settings.*
>
> (Dixon 2017, p5)

So, data is the basis of evidence; using data for improvement can include:

1. using evidence sources and information that are already available (healthcare is awash with data that is not used or employed to full capability, therefore using what is already available should always be the first priority);
2. collating data that is already being generated in practice but is not currently captured or used; or
3. only collecting or generating new information when absolutely necessary.

Data is used to inform various types of evidence. Typically, terms such as 'data' and 'evidence' are associated with empirical research; however, they are equally relevant for audit and quality improvement. The differences and similarities between research, audit and quality improvement were outlined in the Foundations chapter;

however, there is overlap in terms of the data sources, types and sometimes collection and analysis methods.

Sources of evidence

There are multiple and varied sources of evidence that can be used to identify and appraise improvement ideas and potential solutions.

As Elisabeth's story at the start of Part 2 of this book illustrates, she has already reflected on her own experience and observation in practice regarding the challenges and risks to care quality and staff wellbeing associated with giving an effective patient handover. She has also used her previous experience and transferable skills as a journalist to identify a potential solution (i.e. the introduction of a structured handover tool) to enhance the effectiveness of handover in practice. However, Elisabeth is wisely planning to check out her initial ideas by reviewing the published literature on this topic before going any further. This is imperative but there are also other sources of evidence that Elisabeth would be wise to explore at this early stage and completing Activity 4.1 will help you to identify these.

Activity 4.1   Evidence-based practice and research

Take a few minutes to re-read Elisabeth's scenario then make a list of other potential sources of information/data for her to consider.

Or, if you prefer, complete the same activity based on an improvement idea of your own, then discuss the potential sources and types of evidence you identify with your lecturer/ practice supervisor.

Compare your notes with the worked example at the end of this chapter.

The relevant sources and types of data for each improvement topic or idea vary extensively. For example, routine staff/patient surveys yield a lot of very useful data but are unlikely to be specific enough for Elisabeth's needs in the example given, therefore in some cases it can be necessary to collect specific information to inform or evaluate improvement activity. This may be formal, or in the case of quality improvement, informal, for example by seeking feedback from staff on their experiences of handover during a routine team meeting, as part of everyday reflexive practice.

Types of evidence

The type of evidence used to justify an improvement need, a potential solution and ultimately evaluate the effectiveness of an intervention, varies. Depending on the topic and context, the types of evidence may include:

- empirical, peer-reviewed research and evaluation research;
- grey literature such as expert opinion, policy documents, professional guidance and published reports;
- audit reports and data: national and local;
- formal feedback/surveys or consultation data, e.g. from service users, staff and other stakeholders;
- informal or opportunistic feedback, e.g. from service users, staff and other stakeholders.

In addition, the type of data may be quantitative (primarily numbers and equations based), qualitative (primarily words or themes based) or a mixture of both; with varying emphasis on the number of respondents, measurement versus perceptions or cause and effect for example.

Box 4.1   The value of analysing a practice issue: theatre trolleys

Staff were under pressure to increase the throughput of patients in a general theatre's suite. Delays were often experienced due to a lack of trolleys. The team's initial response was to develop an application for capital funding to buy additional trolleys, but they decided to investigate further first. Completing an inventory of the theatre trolley stock indicated that they had more than enough trolleys, but a high proportion were currently unusable. The team's investigation indicated various reasons for this, including some trolleys that needed repair. Thus, they set about addressing these issues rather than seeking additional funding and as a result, experienced a significant drop in the number of delays caused by a trolley not being available when needed.

Identifying improvement-based solutions and evaluating potential options

Analysing the issue and identifying potential solutions

It can be very tempting, and sometimes relatively easy, to immediately identify a change idea or potential solution when you see a need for improvement – however, this is to be resisted! Although ultimately the initial idea or obvious solution may be the one tested, it is crucial to keep an open mind at this stage. Shella's comments at the opening to this chapter illustrate this as she seems to have decided providing health promotion leaflets is the best solution, without apparently considering other options. Systematic consideration of all the factors involved and analysis of the relevant data is the best way to ensure all relevant potential solutions are considered and that any decisions are based on empirical evidence. This process of exploration and clarification also provides a sound basis from which to build support for any proposed change, not only in terms of the information generated but also through involving the relevant stakeholders in this analysis that will underpin any resulting improvement activity.

Many frameworks and tools are available for you to use to support the analysis of practice and service outcomes, especially when a need for improvement is clear. You may already be familiar with the Root Cause Analysis (RCA) approach, which, though attracting increasing critique, remains commonly used by organisations when investigating reported incidents or near misses (Nicolini et al, 2011). A range of tools can support the identification of root causes. For example, the '5 Whys?' is a relatively simple, very commonly used tool to support a basic review of simple problems. It involves writing down the issue at hand, then repeatedly asking 'why?' until the root cause of an issue is identified, enabling potential solutions to be developed. However, the 5 Why's has been criticised as too simplistic when compared to other tools such as a 'tree diagram' (Card, 2017) which are more likely to identify a wider range of issues. For more complex issues, the 5 Whys can be combined with other methods, such as an Ishikawa (cause and effect) diagram (Wong et al, 2016). First developed by organisational theorist Kaoru Ishikawa, this is commonly known as a Fishbone diagram as the elements resemble the skeletal structure of a fish. In this case, starting with the problem statement at the 'head' of the fish, the main categories of causes related to that problem are identified (main branches) and then the 5 Why's can be used to help identify the root causes for each main branch. It is important to use data to explain or justify each aspect of the Ishikawa diagram from the problem statement to each 'bone' of the fish. It can be helpful to start by considering generic categories such as: equipment, people (i.e. manpower, skills etc.), materials, measurement, environment for example. This prompts the team to think about issues with the system that lead to the topic being addressed, avoiding the temptation of blaming people or groups of people.

These are just examples of the tools you can use to analyse the practice problem you want to address or excellent practice you want to replicate and spread. You will find others in most improvement resource toolkits (see the further reading section at the end of this chapter). It is important to remember, however, to always use data when determining the problem statement and each of the causative factors. This data can be quantitative/numerical, but as we saw in Chapter 1, Activity 1.6 can also be from taking notice of what goes on around you during your everyday work and/or comments from colleagues or people accessing services.

Environmental analysis

Appropriate analysis of the local and wider context is a crucial aspect of any successful improvement work. This process is commonly known as an 'environmental analysis' or 'situational analysis' and is particularly important in terms of assessing readiness for change. Various tools can be used to ensure a systematic and comprehensive approach. Some, e.g. SWOT (Strengths, Weaknesses, Opportunities, Threats) or SWOC (Strengths, Weaknesses, Opportunities and Challenges) you may already be very familiar with. These are more generic and can be applied to internal or external assessment. SWOT is best combined with more specific frameworks that are designed to help identify relevant external (e.g. PESTLE) and internal (e.g. McKinsey 7S) factors to be considered regarding your chosen issue to enable a comprehensive analysis. Complete Activity 4.2 now to increase your familiarity with these commonly used tools.

Activity 4.2   Measuring

Take a few minutes to look at a brief overview of two frameworks that are commonly used to inform an environmental analysis before instigating change:

1.   PESTLE: PESTLE analysis – YouTube;
2.   McKinsey 7S: https://www.pocketbook.co.uk/blog/2012/02/28/on-competition-internal-forces-and-the-7-s-model/ (McKInsey 7Ss).

Completing an environmental/readiness for change analysis may indicate, for example, that despite the need for a specific improvement being clear from the data, other factors, e.g. competing priorities or low morale following a previously unsuccessful change, may mean that it would be inadvisable to take forward a certain improvement at a particular point in time. This does not mean the idea should be abandoned altogether but other interventions or external change may be necessary before there can be any chance of it succeeding.

Force Field Analysis can also be useful for assessing readiness for change. You may find it helpful to review Chapter 3, where Lewin's (1951) theory of change was introduced. This involves the identification of driving and resisting forces relevant to the change being considered, along with their relative strengths. The analysis can be focused on the team, departmental, organisation or sector/societal level. Figure 4.1 provides an example of the application of this tool to Elisabeth's situation.

Some key points to consider when using Force Field Analysis are:

- increasing driving forces may seem attractive but result in an increase in resisting forces; the equilibrium does not change but is maintained under increased tension;
- to effect change it is preferable to reduce resisting forces to allow movement toward the desired state without increasing tension;
- driving forces are not necessarily 'positive' as resisting forces are not necessarily 'negative';
- Force Field Analysis is about *perceptions* so requires inclusion (i.e. a broad, outward-facing perspective) by involving wider stakeholders and careful listening;
- the means identified for dealing with resisting forces need to be creative.

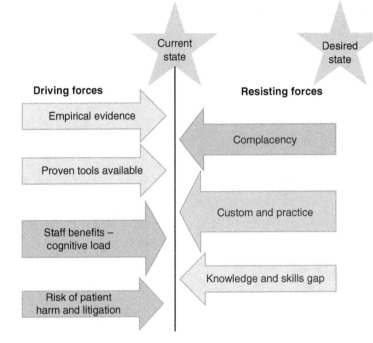

Figure 4.1 Example Force Field Analysis for the introduction of a structured nursing handover tool

The final tool we will consider here in terms of analysing the issue is a driver diagram. These are increasingly used by teams to help develop and depict their working theory about what 'drives' or contributes to the achievement of an improvement aim. A driver diagram demonstrates visually the relationship between three main groups of factors: the primary (or key) drivers that directly contribute to achieving a project aim, secondary drivers (components of the primary drivers) and potential change ideas to test relating to each secondary driver. This is useful for enabling a shared understanding among the core improvement team but also provides a useful tool when communicating with a range of wider stakeholders for any given improvement project (see Chapter 5 for an example of how Harry might use a driver diagram when progressing his change idea).

Generating potential solutions or improvement intervention ideas

Having identified then analysed an excellent aspect of practice you want to spread or an issue to be addressed, the next step is to identify potential solutions or interventions for testing. The aim here is to be as open as possible, to generate a wide range of ideas. Many tools can support this process; we introduce just two here: brainstorming and the 'Z Technique'. You may already be very familiar with brainstorming as a commonly used, creative problem-solving approach in which individuals or small groups contribute their ideas for potential solutions in response to the identified topic or problem.

Options appraisal

As we learned earlier, forging ahead with a single solution without having considered alternative options must be avoided if you want to maximise the chances of success. This is where evaluating each potential solution, also known as options appraisal, is important – it is also normally a requirement of any business case. However, we first need to organise the large number of ideas it is likely we will generate. An Affinity Diagram is often used at this stage to group ideas into categories (commonly 3–6 categories) so that similar ideas can be considered together. Complete Activity 4.3 for further information on how to develop an Affinity Diagram and other stages of the project cycle in which this tool might be useful.

Activity 4.3   Building knowledge

Access this step-by-step guide to Improvement Science, which explains how to develop and when to use an Affinity Diagram and the other stages of a project where it might be useful:

https://www.cec.health.nsw.gov.au/__data/assets/pdf_file/0010/445447/Improvement-Science-Step-by-Step-Guide.pdf

---

Determining which change ideas to take forward and in which order

Dot voting is a common method of agreeing priorities within a group. Each participant is given a number of tokens (dots) and places these against the options they think should be prioritised and those with the most dots or 'votes' are taken forward. One disadvantage of this method is that individuals' priorities may not be based on explicit or shared criteria. Being systematic in how individual ideas are appraised is important so that the merits of each against the project aim are considered. Some ideas may need clarifying, e.g. what exactly would be tested and how, then each can be considered in terms of pre-identified criteria. NHS Scotland proposes using a simple 2x2 prioritisation matrix for this (see Figure 4.2) based on:

- Effort – *Ease of implementation (easy or hard)*, e.g. how costly will it be? can it be tested relatively soon? how long will it take to test – hours, weeks, months? will many people need to be retrained? are those affected likely to welcome the idea and why?; and
- Impact – in terms of *the aim (high or low)*, e.g. how much will the change idea affect the problem? what will be the effect on outcomes? what other indirect effects might there be?

A collaborative approach to this process, involving key stakeholders, helps generate buy-in and increases the likelihood of successful intervention because key groups have participated in the prioritisation process. A step-by-step guide to the process is included in the additional resources section at the end of the chapter but, in summary, each idea is written on a post-it note and placed on the chart, with the group deciding where this should be. This can be done quite quickly and the final results refined through group discussion. Once completed you should be able to see the priorities towards the upper half of the matrix, with the 'quick wins' (lower effort and greater impact) toward the top left. This options appraisal can then be used to inform subsequent prioritisation of the ideas generated, i.e. just because an idea is assessed as hard to implement this does not necessarily mean it should be low priority if the likely impact is great. Free electronic whiteboard software, e.g. Padlet or Miro, can also be used to facilitate this process in a virtual format.

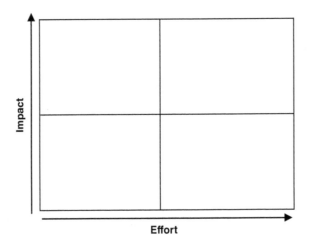

Figure 4.2 Prioritisation matrix

The 'Z Technique' combines a more structured approach to ideas generation with options appraisal and is designed to ensure all sides of the issue and different types of solution are considered. Based on psychological theory, this technique, created by Isabel Myers and further developed by Gordon Lawrence, uses preferences from the Myers-Briggs Type Indicator™ or MBTI™. It can be used to guide individuals and groups through a structured approach to creative problem-solving to ensure consideration of a wide range of options. It can therefore be useful for supporting the application of Part 1 of the MFI and Figure 4.3 provides an overview of an adaptation of this technique. The 'S' and 'N' in the model are used to depict different ways individuals prefer to take in information. 'S' tends to pay attention to what they perceive through their senses: seeing, hearing, touching, smelling and tasting, paying attention to detail, facts and what is real. 'N' on the other hand, tends to pay attention to their 'sixth sense' – or 'gut reaction' – which is driven by an unseen world of meanings, inferences, hunches, insights and connections, focusing more on information in terms of what could be, theoretical possibilities and novelty. The 'T' and 'F' elements of the model depict different preferences for decision-making. 'T' prefers to base decisions on impartial criteria, cause–effect reasoning, constant principles or truths, and logic. 'F' on the other hand prefers making decisions based on values, person-centred criteria and seeking harmony. All preferences have equal value and refer to preferred ways of operating rather than ability; however, considering and planning for individual preferences as guided by this model can be very effectively used when considering how to engage others in the change process. Further information is provided in the further reading section at the end of this chapter.

Whichever techniques are used to generate potential ideas and appraise potential solutions, the key is to involve all the stakeholders in the process. This will ensure the widest possible range of ideas is generated for testing and promotes buy-in from key individuals and groups for the identified change.

Activity 4.4   Critical thinking

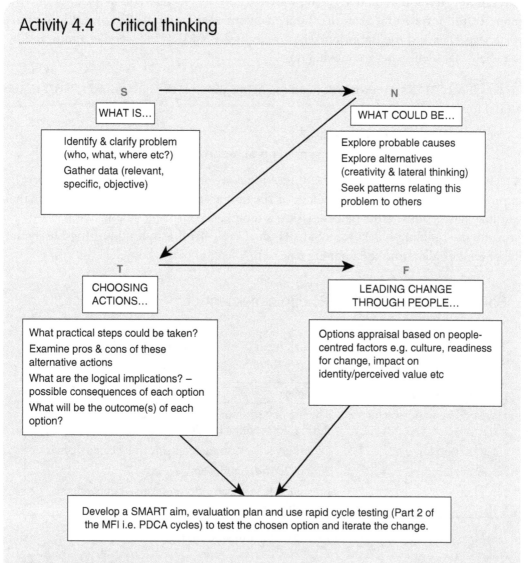

Figure 4.3 The 'Z' Technique

(Continued)

(Continued)

Get together a small group of peers or work colleagues and use the Z Technique outlined in Figure 4.3 to generate as many potential solutions to your chosen practice issue as possible. Remember, your chosen issue need not necessarily be a problem to be fixed but could focus on how to spread an element of good practice. Once this is completed, use the 2x2 prioritisation matrix in Figure 4.2 to agree as a group one solution to test.

Scoping a sustainable improvement idea

Determining the scope of any improvement can mean the difference between success and failure. Developing and agreeing with stakeholders a clear aim helps to define the scope of the improvement effort, hence why we spent time in Chapter 2 looking at what SMART is and the importance of developing a SMART aim, so take a minute now to review that section before moving on.

To develop a SMART aim you will need to answer the first two questions in Part 1 of the Model for Improvement:

- what are we trying to accomplish?
- how will we know that change represents an improvement?

A clear aim statement is also a useful tool for convincing other people to support the improvement – it is part of your 'elevator pitch' – a strategy for influencing others that you may have come across before. Using a template consisting of four basic questions provides the building blocks for a SMART aim; Table 4.1 illustrates this using Elisabeth's improvement idea from the opening part of this section of the book.

Box 4.2 Elisabeth's SMART aim statement

Elisabeth developed her SMART aim statement in two stages. She started by completing the Aim Statement Template below with the help of her practice assessor:

Prompt question	Response
What do we want to achieve?	The use of a structured communication tool by nurses during shift change handovers
Where/who for?	On Primrose Unit, at each nursing shift change handover
How much?	80% of all shift handovers
By when?	June 2022 [use a realistic target date – improvement inevitably takes longer than people anticipate]

Table 4.1 Developing Elisabeth's SMART aim statement

The second stage was to turn the answers to the four questions in the template into an aim statement:

Our aim is that a structured communication tool will be used by nurses during 80% of all shift change handovers on Primrose Unit by June 2022.

It can be tempting, especially if you have a particular solution in mind and are zealous about the 'S' of SMART, to name your chosen solution in the aim statement. Generally, you should try to avoid this because it could be that your original solution is not the best option in practice. Elisabeth has noted this advice and used the more general 'structured communication tool' terminology in her aim. While at the start of her idea she thought the SBAR (Situation, Background, Assessment, Recommendation) tool would be the best solution, she can now appreciate that SBAR is only one of many such tools, so by using this broader term she is not limited to SBAR if this is not the one that is found to work best in her practice context.

Activity 4.5 Critical thinking

Copy a blank version of the template Elisabeth used in Table 4.1, then complete it based on an improvement idea you've identified from your own practice experience; then develop a SMART aim statement from the responses as Elisabeth did. Share this with your practice assessor or peers for feedback.

Further examples of how to use this approach to developing a SMART aim can be found in this short video: https://www.youtube.com/watch?v=rWcV7IE8g2U

Answering the prompts to develop an aim statement for your improvement initiative and using the SMART approach requires some scoping of your improvement. This includes being very clear about what will not be included or achieved as well as what can be expected. Factors to consider when determining the scope of any improvement activity include but are not limited to:

- readiness for change in the target area and/or team members (the findings from the environmental analysis discussed earlier will act as a guide here);
- available resources, e.g. people, equipment, knowledge and skills;
- equipment needed (if relevant).

For example, Elisabeth scoped her aim to include just one clinical area, i.e. Primrose Unit. Some of the factors that influenced this decision are likely to have included for example:

- she had some influence in this setting as it was the placement area she was working in;
- she had discussed the idea with her practice assessor who thought the team would be open to it and willing to help test;
- the initiative would not require any special equipment or resources.

Establishing the scope of any improvement activity, as well as determining the best solution, are crucial aspects of ensuring the change is not only successful but also sustainable. Many projects only succeed because a certain set of circumstances prevail but are not sustained when these change. Addressing the sustainability of any change throughout, beginning right at the start of the improvement process, i.e. during the options appraisal, helps prevent people and systems reverting back to the status quo even following a successful change intervention. As we saw in Chapter 3, Lewin (1951) calls this stage of the change process 'refreezing'.

Sustainability

The sustainability of an improvement is said to have been achieved when a new way of working or a particular outcome becomes the norm or 'business as usual'. There is little point in making any positive change unless it can be sustained in the long term. In fact, introducing a successful change that cannot be sustained can have a detrimental impact as it raises staff or service user expectations that cannot then be maintained. It is therefore crucial that the sustainability of any proposed improvement is considered during the early stages of development. Addressing sustainability is closely connected to scoping an improvement. For example, it is unlikely that Elisabeth could ensure a structured communication tool is used for all nursing shift-change handovers in every clinical area in her organisation, so aiming to achieve this in just one area initially offers a much better chance of making the change 'stick' or become part of everyday practice there, before seeking to spread the change to other areas. A very useful tool to help us address sustainability when planning an improvement was co-produced with groups of frontline staff, administrative and clinical leaders, academics, improvement experts and individuals with relevant expertise from other industries. This NHS Sustainability Model (Maher et al, 2010) can be used as a diagnostic tool to assess the likelihood of your improvement being sustained by identifying the strengths and weaknesses of your change plan in relation to ten key factors in three main areas. Some considerations in each of these areas include:

- *Staff* – e.g. to what extent have staff been involved in developing the proposed change? Do the staff see the proposed change as an improvement worth sustaining and have any concerns been taken account of? To what extent are senior and clinical leaders involved and 'championing' the initiative? What infrastructure is in place to identify and address staff knowledge and skills gaps in relation to the new way of working?
- *Process* – e.g. how credible is the evidence on which the proposed change is based? Does the change rely on a specific individual or group and can it be sustained if these are removed? Are mechanisms in place to monitor and assess progress?
- *Organisation* – e.g. how well does the proposed improvement align with the organisation's goals, vision and current strategic priorities, values and culture? To what extent does the infrastructure (such as role descriptions) enable the proposed change?

Having assessed the likely sustainability of a proposed improvement, you can then use the NHS Sustainability Guide part of the model as a practical guide for how to increase the chances of sustaining the change in the longer term.

Activity 4.6   Measuring

Access the NHS Sustainability Model template (see the further reading section at the end of this chapter). Answer the prompt questions in the three areas then add the scores for each and plot them on the Master Score page; then add them together to produce your Sustainability Total Score. You can then plot this information on the portal (spider) diagram and/or the bar chart template to identify potential areas in which sustainability might be improved. You should then review the Sustainability Guide (see the further reading section at the end of this chapter) for practical tips on how to address the aspects of the improvement the sustainability assessment highlights as potential areas for enhancement and amend your plan accordingly. Discuss this assessment with your practice assessor and/or peers.

The role of evaluation and measurement planning

The importance of planning how you will evaluate whether any improvement actually results in positive change and identifying the appropriate measures you will use for this was introduced in earlier chapters. There we considered the need to include planning for evaluation of any improvement activity as a core part of the initial design, rather than a later 'add on' as is often the case. Evaluation is particularly important for supporting sustainable improvement. This is one of the advantages of using the MFI (Langley et al, 2009) to guide any improvement because the measurement/evaluation data from each rapid test PDCA cycle not only helps determine the effectiveness of each iteration or 'tweak', but crucially also helps to build real-time evidence regarding the impact of the change as it progresses. Where negative effects are identified, this can prevent waste, which might include time and other resources, but also minimises risk as any negative impact is determined early. Where positive, evaluation data can be used to support a future expansion or a business case for wider application of the change.

The Seven Steps to Measurement for Improvement (NHS England/Improvement, online) provide a structure and method to support the development of effective measures in practice. After defining the aim (Step 1), choosing and defining your measures (Steps 2 and 3) must be completed before the collection of any data.

Using a range of different types of measures maximises the comprehensiveness of the evaluation. As we learned in Chapter 2, any change in one area of a complex adaptive system like healthcare invariably has an impact on others. Therefore, as well as using outcome and process measures to determine what the outcomes of the improvement and experiences of the process of change and new way of working are, wider impact in the system can be determined by the judicious use of balance measures. This enables identification of any unintended consequences. For example, if the assessment of patients likely to require an x-ray is streamlined and made more efficient in A&E, this may create a backlog in the radiology department that will have a detrimental effect on the patient experience overall and will not support effective collaboration between departments if not considered, and the radiology department staff consulted, before the change is made. This serves as an important reminder of the importance of identifying and involving all the key stakeholders, as we discussed in the Introduction chapter and have developed in subsequent chapters. If you are unsure of what an outcome, process or balance measure is, you should review the 'measuring for improvement' section in Chapter 2 now before moving on to complete the activity below, where you will put this knowledge into practice. Ensuring that you make measurement part of the normal work routine and wherever possible, using data and data collection systems that already exist, will improve the chances of data being collected reliably and sustainably by reducing the burden on staff.

When considering the relevant measures for your improvement, you will need to consider what data you will collect for each measure and how. The sources of evaluation data and the methods used to collect and analyse it can be similar to those used for research, but their use in the context of improvement is different. You may find it helpful to review the 'Differentiating quality improvement from audit and research' section in the Foundations chapter as a reminder of these differences before moving on.

Activity 4.7 Measuring

You are a member of the team helping Elisabeth to progress her improvement idea to introduce a structured patient handover. Fill in the template below by identifying at least one measure for each of the categories that you would suggest she uses – you can add extra lines! Discuss your ideas with your peers and practice assessor or lecturer.

A worked example is provided at the end of the chapter for you to review after completing this activity.

Type of measure	What will you measure?	Why did you choose this measure? How will it help you determine whether or not the change is an improvement?	What data will you collect and how?
Outcome			
Process			
Balance			

Chapter summary

This chapter has introduced some key considerations and commonly used tools to enable you to identify and develop an evidence-based, contextualised and sustainable improvement idea of relevance to practice. In doing so it has built on concepts introduced in earlier chapters such as the complexity of healthcare, involving and working with others, designing sustainable improvement and the role of measurement and evaluation throughout the improvement process. This chapter has focused primarily on how to apply Part 1 (i.e. the three questions) of the Model for Improvement (Langley et al, 2009):

1. What are we trying to accomplish?
2. How will we know that change represents an improvement?
3. What changes can we make that will lead to improvement?

and has introduced you to a range of tools that are commonly used to support this. Completing the suggested activities and using the worked examples at the end of the chapter has enabled you to experience applying the chapter content to your own improvement idea or Elisabeth's situation. The following chapter will focus in more detail on evaluation as a core aspect of any improvement activity.

Glossary

Scope: concerns the extent of something. Establishing clear aims and objectives helps to establish the scope of any endeavour as they can be used to determine clear boundaries regarding what will be excluded as well as what will be included.

CQC: the Care Quality Commission is the independent regulator for health and social care in England. Other nations have similar bodies. Examples include: RQIA (Regulation and Quality Improvement Authority, Northern Ireland); the Care Inspectorate (Scotland and Wales); Commission on Safety and Quality in Health Care (Australia); US Department of Health and Human Services (HHS); Office of the Inspector General (OIG); Norwegian Board of Health Supervision.

Business Case: structured document succinctly laying out, for an intended audience of approvers and/or funders, the evidence-informed rationale, justification and details of a proposed practice or service improvement.

Answers to activities

Activity 4.1 Evidence-based practice and research

Additional sources of information Elisabeth might use to inform her handover improvement idea might include:

- *Friends and family data* – is there any learning from recent friends and family reports that involves the handover process/effectiveness?

- *Audit data* – is there a recent handover audit and what were the findings/recommendations made?
- *Complaints and compliments data* – is handover a factor in any recent complaints or compliments and what might this tell us?
- *Adverse Events and near miss data* – is handover a contributory factor associated with any of these? If so, in what way?
- *Clinical outcomes data*, e.g. safety thermometer
- CQC *reports* – is there anything in recent CQC reports relating to handover? – this may be most likely found in the 'safe' or 'effective' standards sections
- *National safety alerts* – have there been any recent safety alerts associated with patient handover practices?

Activity 4.7. Measuring

Type of measure	What will you measure?	Why did you choose this measure? How will it help you determine whether or not the change is an improvement?	What data will you collect and how?
Outcome	Number and/or percentage of shift handovers in which the structured communication tool was used	To determine the extent to which the project aim (i.e. tool used in 80% of all handovers) has been met	Project lead (or designated colleague) keep tally chart of whether or not structured handover tool was used at each shift change.
Process	Staff views on the new-style handovers e.g. - How easy to use? - Anything unclear? - Do the sections make sense, are they fit for purpose/usable? - How easy is the relevant handover paperwork (eg SBAR) pad to find? How often is it missing/empty?	To determine how the format and other characteristics of the new style handover are working for those involved. This will enable adjustments to be made that will support staff engagement with the change and to what extent it is sustained over time to become normal handover practice.	**What:** verbal staff comments and views on their experiences of using the tool and/or being in a handover when it is used. Notes from tally chart of contextual factors that promoted/enabled or prevented use of structured handover tool. **When/how:** (1) during weekly team meeting (arrange to agenda 5-10min discussion); (2) opportunistically – staff can provide email/ verbal comments to project lead on an ad hoc basis.
Balance	Number and type of queries from colleagues seeking more patient information or clarification after the handover	This will indicate if the all the relevant information is being included in the handover.	Staff feedback on the frequency and types of additional information sought by colleagues post handover and potential causes of this.

Type of measure	What will you measure?	Why did you choose this measure? How will it help you determine whether or not the change is an improvement?	What data will you collect and how?
	Any untoward incidents or near misses associated with missing handover information involving the new-style handover process?	Handover is a crucial and complex clinical activity that has significant implications for patient safety and quality of care. Measures will therefore be needed to check that the new handover process does not lead to increased risk.	Routinely collected serious untoward incident (SUI)/near miss data.

Useful websites

https://www.bhf.org.uk/informationsupport/publications/healthcare-and-innovations/business-case-toolkit--template# British Heart Foundation – Business Case Toolkit – Includes a business case checklist/template.

https://www.imperial.ac.uk/media/imperial-college/administration-and-support-services/staff-development/public/impex/Decision-making-using-MBTI.pdf; MBTI® Z model and decision-making https://collegiategateway.com/improve-your-decision-making-use-the-zig-zag-model/

https://learn.nes.nhs.scot/3138/quality-improvement-zone/qi-tools/measurement-plan Measurement Plan Template and further information

https://www.england.nhs.uk/sustainableimprovement/qsir-programme/qsir-tools/ NHS Quality Improvement Toolkit – access to a wide range of improvement tools.

https://www.england.nhs.uk/improvement-hub/wp-content/uploads/sites/44/2017/11/NHS-Sustainability-Guide-2010.pdf NHS Sustainability Guide

https://www.england.nhs.uk/wp-content/uploads/2021/03/qsir-sustainability-model.pdf NHS Sustainability Model

https://www.pocketbook.co.uk/blog/2012/02/28/on-competition-internal-forces-and-the-7-s-model/ 7S Framework

https://www.england.nhs.uk/wp-content/uploads/2021/03/qsir-pareto.pdf Pareto analysis A simple way of determining the issues with the greatest potential for improvement based on relative frequency or size. It is based on the 80/20 rule that in a given situation 80% of effects come from 20% of the causes.

https://learn.nes.nhs.scot/ Prioritisation Matrix – Step-by-step guide to using a Prioritisation Matrix Access to quality improvement resources and training

https://www.publichealth.hscni.net/directorates/health-and-social-care-quality-improvement Health and Social Care Quality Improvement Northern Ireland

https://www.healthcareimprovementscotland.org/ Healthcare Improvement Scotland

https://www.england.nhs.uk/improvement-hub/ NHS England Improvement Hub

https://www.england.nhs.uk/improvement-hub/wp-content/uploads/sites/44/2017/11 NHS-Sustainability-Model-2010.pdf NHS Sustainability Model

https://heiw.nhs.wales/education-and-training/dental/quality-improvement/ Quality Improvement Wales

Chapter 5

Planning and implementing improvement

Catherine Delves-Yates and Claire Brockwell

NMC Future Nurse: Standards of Proficiency for Registered Nurses

This chapter will address the following platforms and proficiencies:

Platform 1: Being an accountable professional

1.1 understand and act in accordance with the Code: Professional standards of practice and behaviour for nurses, midwives and nursing associates, and fulfil all registration requirements.

Platform 6: Improving safety and quality of care

6.4 demonstrate an understanding of the principles of improvement methodologies, participate in all stages of audit activity and identify appropriate quality improvement strategies.
6.9 work with people, their families, carers and colleagues to develop effective improvement strategies for quality and safety, sharing feedback and learning from positive outcomes and experiences, mistakes and adverse outcomes and experiences.
6.11 acknowledge the need to accept and manage uncertainty, and demonstrate an understanding of strategies that develop resilience in self and others.

Chapter aims

After reading this chapter you should be able to:

- apply the MFI **methodology** to a selected quality improvement idea of relevance to your role;
- develop a realistic project plan and monitoring framework using appropriate tools and frameworks;
- apply the principles of stakeholder management when developing a project outline and implementation plan;
- identify potential unforeseen challenges for quality improvements in practice and strategies to manage these.

From my experience in my last placement, I think I have a good idea that would improve the care of the people I nursed. I also have some thoughts of how my idea could work in practice, but I don't have a coherent plan. What do I?

(Maeve, registered nurse, community)

I am confused! I have been told I need to use a model to implement my improvement idea, but there are so many models for so many different things! Why should I use a model, and which one should I choose?

(Richard, 2nd year children's nursing student)

Introduction

Our role as nurses is exciting, extending from being responsible for delivering effective one-to-one interventions to the people we nurse and their loved ones, to influencing how best to meet the health needs of whole populations. Quality improvement is a cornerstone of nursing, all healthcare organisations expect nurses not just to deliver safe and effective care, but also to work with service users/carers and colleagues to improve the quality of that care. As demonstrated by Maeve and Richard, who we met at the start of this chapter, nurses and other healthcare professionals are in a prime position to make improvements in the quality of services by identifying and testing out ideas.

Previous chapters have introduced you to a wide range of methods, tools and approaches designed to support the planning and implementation of quality improvement ideas. In this chapter we will help you develop your understanding of how what you have read can be applied in practice to translate an improvement idea into real life. As Maeve and Richard highlight at the start of this chapter, even when you have developed an improvement idea, there are still choices to be made and further thinking to do about how you will manage and implement it.

The chances of a change being effectively adopted in practice are greatly increased if you apply a systematic approach to its implementation. Preceding chapters have introduced the systematic approach we will use here. We will now focus on applying the explanatory version of the Model for Improvement (MFI) introduced in the Foundations chapter to help you develop a realistic and dynamic plan for implementing improvement. This will include you using project management skills to devise a monitoring framework for the change, to ensure you remain 'on track' to achieve the aims identified in a timely fashion. Monitoring progress is an important aspect of any quality improvement, as in everyday life we frequently meet challenges, some of which are expected. It is, however, also possible that we may meet unforeseen challenges, so we will also consider and discuss strategies for managing these.

Throughout this book it has been made very clear that to effectively implement an improvement, we not only need to work strategically and systematically, following a model, but must also include all relevant stakeholders at every stage. In this chapter we will therefore apply the principles of stakeholder management to our improvement planning.

The value of project management skills

Just as leadership and management skills are important to all nursing students and registered nurses, project management skills are valuable because they are a systematic way of methodically breaking tasks down to make them achievable. Nurses use project management all the time as they oversee all the 'mini-projects' needed to care for people effectively, such as the planning, negotiation and organisation skills required to help a person walk to the washroom and take a shower for the first time after an operation. This fundamental care activity shares many of the skills required to manage a larger, formal project. The structures, models and processes of project management, which are often called tools, were originally created in business and manufacturing to clearly define tasks and processes, making them easy to replicate to ensure quality (Weaver, 2007). By using these techniques to introduce and manage quality improvement-related change in healthcare we can ensure each step is organised to help achieve the desired aims, goals and outcomes efficiently (Collins, 2018).

Activity 5.1   Reflection

Before we delve further into planning and implementation of a quality improvement, we need to step back to review the 'bigger picture'. As highlighted in preceding chapters, the importance of quality improvement and the fact that nurses are responsible for change and innovation in nursing are clearly evident in the Code (NMC, 2018b) and the 'Future Nurse: standards of proficiencies for registered nurses' (NMC, 2018a).

Review these two documents and consider

- What stimulated your desire to change the current situation?
- How are you fulfilling the Code and the 'Future Nurse' proficiencies?

Write down your thoughts. It may be useful to share these thoughts with others involved in the change as they represent the factors motivating you to improve nursing practice.

Why use a quality improvement model?

We use models in many areas of nursing to ensure that we work in a systematic fashion. For example, we frequently apply a model to guide our reflections, to help us focus on learning from experience, develop self-awareness and avoid simply retelling what happened. Reflective models give our writing structure, increase the analytical depth and guide us through the process of reflection (Delves-Yates, 2021). There is, however, no 'best' or 'right' reflective model; you need to choose the one that feels most comfortable for you and helps you learn from your experience. The same applies to using quality improvement models. There are many models, which are also sometimes referred to as theories, frameworks or tools. Terms like these simply mean that they are structures, templates or guides to help you to achieve an aim or task. All models will help you create order in a quality improvement and effectively manage change, increasing the likelihood of positive results. As discussed in Chapters 1 and 3, among the most frequently applied models in healthcare quality improvement are the Model for Improvement (MFI) (Langley et al, 2009), Kotter's 8 step model of managing change (Kotter, 2012), Lewin's 3 step model, which focuses on the psychology of change (Lewin, 1951) and the NHS Change Model Guide (2018). Similarly, models devised to help manage projects are often used, for example the Six Stage Project Management Guide (NHSIII, 2010) and Bridges Transition Model (Bridges, 1986), which focuses upon the personal and human aspects of change. Table 5.1 illustrates how some common models can be applied to improvement, either individually or combined.

Planning and implementing change using the explanatory Model for Improvement (MFI)

Throughout this book we focus on the explanatory MFI to guide you through the improvement process in practice. To briefly revise what has previously been said, the MFI was specifically developed to support the development of small-scale and sustainable change in circumstances where the impetus for change arises from those engaged in the situation. This is exactly the position nurses and other healthcare professionals frequently find themselves in, thus making the MFI especially relevant for guiding practitioner-led improvement.

Models

Project management	Change			Quality improvement	Transition
Six stage project management guide	NHS Change Model	Kotter 8 steps	Lewin	The Explanatory Model for Improvement	Bridges' Transition Model
1. Start out Identify the service to be improved Explain the aim of the planned change Highlight the rationale for the change	Our shared purpose Leadership by all System drivers	**Creating the climate for change** 1. Create urgency 2. Form a powerful coalition 3. Create a vision for change	**Unfreeze** Determine what needs to change Ensure there is strong leadership support Create the need for change Manage and understand the doubts and concerns	What are we trying to accomplish? (set the aim) How will we know that a change is an improvement? (select measures)	**Ending, losing, letting go** Resistance to the change initiative Uncertainty and fear Emotional upheaval
2. Define and scope Outline the objectives of the change as measurable targets Identify the key individuals who are critical to achieving the service improvement proposal 3. Measure and understand Explain how you are going to establish pre-change measurements for the objectives identified in stage 2	Motivate and mobilise	**Engage and enable the organisation** 4. Communicate the vision 5. Empower action 6. Create quick wins	**Change** Communicate often Dispel rumours Empower action Involve people in the process	What change can we make that will result in an improvement? (develop ideas for change)	**Neutral zone** Resentment towards the change initiative Low morale and low productivity Anxiety about their role or identity Scepticism about the change initiative

Models

Project management	Change			Quality improvement	Transition
Six stage project management guide	**NHS Change Model**	**Kotter 8 steps**	**Lewin**	**The Explanatory Model for Improvement**	**Bridges' Transition Model**
4. Design and plan Produce an 'action plan' outlining the tasks required to achieve the change.	Improvement tools. Measurement Project performance	**Implementing and sustaining for change** 7. Build the change		P – Plan it D – Do it C – Check the results	**The new beginning** Acceptance, people have begun to embrace the change initiative.
5. Pilot and implement Identify the leadership approach to be adopted in the implementation of the change. How can change management be used to assist the implementation of the change?					
6. Sustain and share How will you know that the change has been successful? How will you ensure that new ways of working are sustained? How will you share the improvement with colleagues and other practice areas?	and management	8. Make it stick	**Refreeze** Anchor the changes to the culture Develop ways to sustain the change Provide support and training Celebrate successes	A – Act depending upon what is learnt	High energy Openness to learning Renewed commitment to the group or their role

Table 5.1 Integrating models for project management, change, quality improvement and transition

One advantage of using the MFI is that evaluation data is generated as soon as you start to implement the improvement idea and is then used to guide the next steps. This reduces risk and potential waste of resources on good change ideas that are just not viable. Used appropriately, the MFI offers a rigorous, experimental approach to improvement, addressing complex problems and responding to the unforeseen impact of change (Reed and Card, 2016). Therefore, it is unsurprising that the MFI is commonly used to promote sustainable change not only in UK healthcare settings, but also internationally.

Applying the MFI involves the testing and modification of a new idea before it is widely implemented. This process of repetitive testing has two major benefits. First, it reduces the risk of negative outcomes from working in a new way, so the safety of those receiving care and the quality of that care is ensured. Second, the approach can promote engagement of those who are uncertain of the value of an improvement idea, because evidence against intended outcomes is gathered as it is generated. This evidence can be used to either demonstrate that the improvement is worth pursuing, or that it needs adaption to ensure that the change introduced achieves what is required.

Within each stage of the MFI a range of tools and techniques is used to support each step of the improvement process. To help you understand how to use a model to plan and implement an improvement we will apply the explanatory version of the original MFI (Langley et al, 2009) explained in the Foundations chapter because the additional information it provides should help you understand how to use the model effectively (see Figure 5.1).

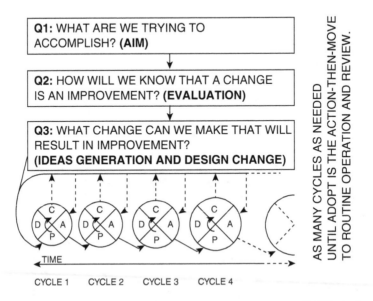

Figure 5.1 Explanatory version of the Model for Improvement (MFI) (adapted from Langley et al, 2009)

As is illustrated in Figure 5.1, the explanatory version of MFI outlines the processes you need to follow to systematically plan and implement an improvement idea. The model has two main parts that are used cyclically. Having just two parts, and the user-friendly language explaining them, makes the explanatory MFI an excellent model to choose. To help you fully understand how to apply this model in practice yourself, we will consider how Harry (from Part 1) and Elisabeth (from Part 2) could use it to plan and implement their ideas. First, we will work through how Harry could apply Part 1 of the explanatory MFI to his idea; then we will consider how Elisabeth could apply Part 2 of the explanatory MFI to her idea.

Table 5.2 provides a quick recap of the idea Harry wants to introduce. See Part 1 for full details.

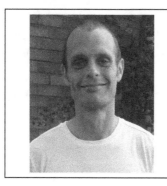

Harry's improvement idea

Organise patient information folders so information is in the same order, with clearly identified sections.

Table 5.2   Quick recap: Harry's improvement

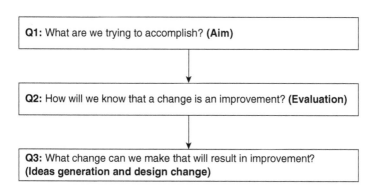

Q1: What are we trying to accomplish? **(Aim)**

Q2: How will we know that a change is an improvement? **(Evaluation)**

Q3: What change can we make that will result in improvement? **(Ideas generation and design change)**

Figure 5.2   Part 1 of the explanatory MFI

Getting started with the MFI ...

The first part of the explanatory MFI (see Figure 5.2) is designed to help you clearly understand the problem to be addressed.

While you may feel you already have this understanding, it is worth investing time to ensure this is the case, because unless you can simply and quickly describe the change you are aiming for, it will be very difficult to convince others of its value. As discussed in previous chapters, introducing change requires a wide range of skills, one of which is the ability to inspire others and convince them of the value of what you wish to achieve. Being able to explain an improvement and the benefit it brings in 30 seconds (see Activity 5.2) is an excellent tactic to employ.

Activity 5.2   Communication

An elevator pitch is a brief (30 seconds) talk outlining the key points of the change. It is called an 'elevator pitch' because it takes approximately the same time as you would spend in an elevator with someone.

It is a challenging but highly effective way to share an idea. Using the prompts identified in Figure 5.3, devise an elevator pitch Harry could use to share his idea in 30 seconds.

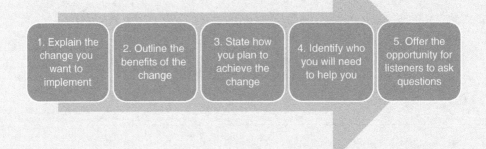

Figure 5.3   5 Step elevator pitch

When you have done this, review the template answer at the end of the chapter for comparison.

When devising a quality improvement, the amount of information you need to consider, organise and share with others can feel overwhelming. You are not alone in feeling this way; even experienced quality improvement practitioners can share your thoughts. Some helpful guidelines you can apply to enable the marshalling of this information are known as SQUIRE 2.0 (see Ogrinc et al, 2016, and further reading at the end of this chapter to view the most recent version).

Continuing our focus on Part 1 of the MFI (Figure 5.2), the three questions it poses are fundamental to developing your improvement idea and understanding what the change in practice is. This sounds very simple but, as you may have found when developing an elevator pitch (Activity 5.2), it can be more complex than you think. Being clear about exactly what you aim to accomplish, how you will know the change has had a positive effect, and precisely what the change you need to make is, involves careful consideration.

To help you do this, the first MFI question,

'What are we trying to accomplish?'

requires setting an improvement aim. Chapter 2 explained 'SMART' aims, so it may be helpful to review the topic by referring to Chapter 2 now. A quality improvement aim is a clear, specific summary of what you want to achieve because of the improvement idea. Harry's improvement aim could be:

For all patient bedside information folders to be organised in a standardised order, with each section clearly labelled.

Thinking of Harry's aim in this way would enable an achievable standard for the presentation of all information folders for the people being cared for in his area to be set. Also, stating his aim in this way will help Harry clearly identify what he wishes the improvement to accomplish, which would help him to explain the idea to others. At this early stage, Harry also needs to consider how to evaluate the change, which identifying a 'SMART' aim will also help with.

The second question in Part 1 of the MFI is,

'How will we know that a change is an improvement?'

This is an equally important question, which may make you scratch your head, as describing this clearly can be deceptively tricky. The thinking you need to do to answer this question is, however, a strength of the MFI. As already emphasised, these questions help you work out how to evaluate the change at this early stage in the development of an improvement idea, by ensuring that you:

- focus upon how you will know what effect the change has;
- generate specific criteria to determine this.

As explained in Chapter 2, Harry is likely to need multiple measures to find out what effect the change has. Thus, his change could be an improvement if

1. healthcare staff report being able to easily find the information they want to access;
2. healthcare staff report that documenting information in the patient information folders is taking less time than prior to the change;

3. when Harry checks a random sample of patient information folders, he will find that at least 50% of them are organised in the agreed order, with each section clearly identified;

4. staff groups are happy with the ordering of the information.

Setting a target of at least 50% for the third criterion may seem surprising, as the change is likely to be more effective if 100% of folders are organised in the new way. It is important, however, to focus on what is reasonable and achievable, especially when first implementing a new way of working. Harry may decide to increase this value later in the change process but setting realistic evaluation criteria is always a priority. In clearly stating these three criteria, Harry now has a tangible way to evaluate or measure the impact of the improvement.

The final question in Part 1 of the MFI asks,

'What change can we make that will result in improvement?'

Focusing again upon Harry's improvement, he needs to think carefully about what he could do to achieve the aim he identified in response to question one. This is a very appropriate point for Harry to thoroughly review his idea for improvement, even if this may seem an unnecessary, backward step. It is often the case that we come up with an initial improvement idea before really having considered exactly what we are aiming to achieve and how we can best translate an idea to practice. We may be certain an initial idea is the perfect solution to the problem we are experiencing, and it may be the case that we have 'stumbled' upon the ideal solution in our first thinking. It is also possible that there is a better solution, or that there are alternative approaches.

An excellent tool to help with this is a driver diagram. As outlined in Chapter 4, a driver diagram demonstrates visually the relationship between three main groups of factors: the primary (or key) drivers that directly contribute to achieving a project aim, secondary drivers (components of the primary drivers) and potential change ideas to test relating to each secondary driver. As is shown by Figure 5.4, a driver diagram could help Harry think critically about and expand his understanding of potential approaches he could apply.

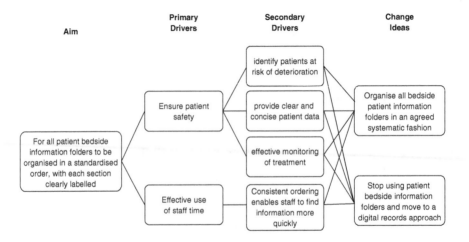

Figure 5.4 Harry's driver diagram

It is only by critically questioning our first thoughts, considering previous practice and reviewing the relevant literature to investigate whether others have effectively solved the same problem, that we can be certain an idea is good. Appraising options and evidence were discussed in Chapter 4, so review the material there for a reminder. As is always the case in healthcare, we must always underpin our actions with rigorous evidence. Thinking very carefully about your idea in light of the evidence supporting it will further help you to develop the ability to explain what you want to change and why. This is an excellent time to use the critical thinking skills developed throughout your studies so far, as applying these here will ensure any change introduced is safe, effective and has the best chance of success.

Activity 5.3   Critical thinking

Preceding chapters and Table 5.1 introduced you to commonly used quality improvement tools and some suggestions for how they can be used to support planning and implementing improvement. If you were Harry, what tools could he use to assist him with applying the first part of the MFI?

Quality improvement tool	At which point of the MFI Part 1 might it be used?
	Initial question 1 – 'What are you trying to accomplish?'
	Initial question 2 – 'How will you know that a change is an improvement?'
	Initial question 3 – 'What change can we make that will result in improvement?'

Table 5.3   Quality improvement tools Harry could use in Part 1 of the MFI

Make a note of your thoughts in the empty column of Table 5.3, then compare these with the sample answer at the end of the chapter.

Part 2 of the explanatory MFI

To help you understand how to apply the second part of the explanatory MFI in practice we will consider how Elisabeth (from Chapter 4) could use it to plan and implement her idea. Table 5.4 provides a quick recap of what Elisabeth wants to introduce (see Part 2 for full details).

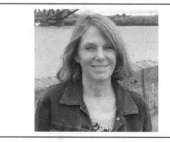

Elisabeth's improvement idea

Introduce a tool which helps nurses to provide an effective handover of patient information.

Table 5.4   Quick recap: Elisabeth's improvement idea

When applying Part 2 of the explanatory MFI (see Figure 5.5) the terms Plan, Do, Check, Act (PDCA) are used rather than the terms Plan, Do, Study, Act (PDSA) that are often applied as we believe they more clearly describe the actions undertaken at each stage. This approach also reflects the original work of Walter Shewart in the 1920s, who devised a Plan, Do, Check, Act cycle (NHS England & NHS Improvement, 2022).

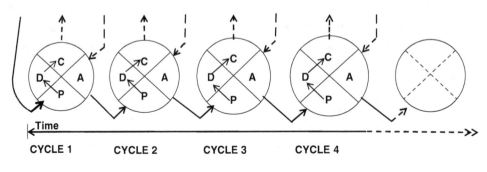

Figure 5.5   Part 2 of the explanatory MFI

Although one of the benefits of the MFI is its simplicity, it is important to remember that this in no way means that achieving successful change is easy. Previous chapters have highlighted the many skills you need to employ when introducing change, with effective and meticulous planning being one of them. Being adaptable is also important because although we will discuss the PDCA stages in order, the process of introducing change in practice may not proceed in such a methodical, linear fashion. It may therefore be necessary to backtrack and reappraise what was originally planned (Connelly, 2021).

Successful change invariably involves multiple PDCA cycles to achieve in tangible sustained improvement, as illustrated in Figure 5.5.

Plan

The first action needed is to assemble a team with the necessary knowledge to bring about the change desired. You need to think carefully about the skills you will need to apply to implement the improvement idea, and who possesses them. Also remember, as discussed in previous chapters, the 'team' needs to include the relevant stakeholders, as their views, experiences and insights are invaluable. As the instigator of change you will be 'heading up the team' but remember this doesn't mean you need to be expert in all areas. The passion you have for the change makes you the correct person to lead it, but the support of a knowledgeable group will be needed for success. Think carefully about who to involve, you may want to work with people who are not only committed to introducing the improvement identified, but are also generally forward thinking, positive and resilient as they will bring these strengths as well as their specific expertise. Do not forget, however, to involve people who are sometimes resistant to change. If you can include them and gain their support, they will also offer a valuable perspective, helping to anticipate problems or overcome resistance. It is also likely that the team needs to represent a range of staff from different disciplines, to reflect the multidisciplinary nature of healthcare. Once the team is assembled, ensure everyone is clear about the roles you will each play, what individual responsibilities are, the time frame involved and set dates for regular progress meetings.

Next, revisit the three questions in Part 1 of the explanatory MFI with the team, including stakeholders. Doing this provides a review of what you want to accomplish, how you will know the change has been an improvement and what the actual change will be. Although you considered these questions at the start, this is another opportunity to check that what you originally thought is still the best course of action. You now also have the benefit of the team, who will bring differing perspectives and are likely to be able to help confirm or further develop the initial responses.

At this stage it is vital to think about the context you are functioning within and the processes you are currently using. An excellent way to do this is for the team to answer the questions outlined in Figure 5.6.

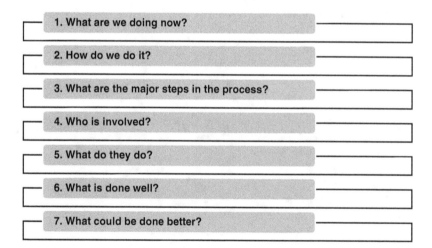

1. What are we doing now?

2. How do we do it?

3. What are the major steps in the process?

4. Who is involved?

5. What do they do?

6. What is done well?

7. What could be done better?

Figure 5.6   Questions to help in 'Plan'

At this point it may also be helpful to perform a SWOT analysis, as discussed in Chapter 4, to help you answer some of the questions in Figure 5.6.

Developing a project plan and monitoring framework

As a nursing student you will already be acutely aware of the value of managing your time and prioritising tasks. Defined simply, project plans and monitoring frameworks are overall plans of what, where, how, by whom and at what cost? Thus, they can be considered as 'the essence of Plan' in every PDCA cycle. Depending upon the reason for the development of an improvement idea and what is required of you for the learning pro-gramme you are undertaking, the issue of funding the change should be considered. This may be purely theoretical, for example if you are required to identify and plan a potential improvement but not implement it in practice. If implementation is required, you may also need to demonstrate the ability to access and manage a budget in practice. Either way, the financial costs involved are likely to be small; aiming for cost-neutral or cost-saving improvement is always the ideal, though funding can be secured where nec-essary if supported by a sound business case (review Chapter 4 for further details).

Project plans were first used in the late 19th century by organisations seeking to achieve comparable high-quality products or services in different departments and sometimes different countries. Project management disciplines evolved with their specific attributes being the ability to describe, manage and control change, because clearly defined techniques used systematically create more replicable and compara-ble outcomes. There are many different approaches to project management, which again involve the application of a specialised range of tools. One tool that is very ben-eficial when planning and implementing an improvement project is a Gantt chart, named after its creator Henry Gantt (1861–1919). This specialised chart is highly effective in visually communicating timescales and displaying a timeline of actions that are broken down into tasks. See Figure 5.7 for an example of a Gantt chart.

Project Start:	Sat, 7/16/2022							
Display Week:	1		Jul 11, 2022		Jul 18, 2022			
			11 12 13 14 15 16 17 18 19 20 21 22 23 24					

TASK	START	END	M T W T F S S M T W T F S S
Identify whether ladder in tights is suitable for darning	7/16/22	7/16/22	
Consult samples of darning wool to locate correct colour	7/16/22	7/17/22	
Buy the correct colour darning wool	7/17/22	7/18/22	
Buy a darning needle	7/17/22	7/17/22	
Buy a thimble	7/17/22	7/17/22	
Thread darning needle with darning wool	7/19/22	7/19/22	
Place thimble on finger	7/19/22	7/19/22	
Turn tights inside out	7/19/22	7/19/22	
Darn ladder in Superman's tights	7/20/22	7/21/22	
Check for further ladders	7/21/22	7/21/22	

Figure 5.7   A Gantt chart: darn Superman's tights

The aim of the Gantt chart in Figure 5.7 is to darn Superman's tights, which probably will not feature highly in many healthcare-related improvement plans, but clearly dem-onstrates that even superheroes must take planning seriously!

As Figure 5.7 shows, a Gantt chart is a visual list of tasks displayed along a timeline. Each task is represented by a horizontal bar, the length of which shows the time estimated for it to take place. The chart indicates the order in which tasks need to be completed. Some tasks run in parallel; others are dependent on each other. The tasks may also list the individuals responsible, although this can make the chart more difficult to read. Including detail on the chart is important however, as this allows all involved to understand when their effort is required and for what, thus enabling efficiency and accountability. Making tasks visual also highlights steps that may have been overlooked and determines the elements critical to the success of the project. Understanding which tasks cannot be started until others are completed and identifying the stages and sequence required make it clear how long all the activities will take from start to finish, which is highly important in effective planning.

Applying the principles of stakeholder management

As considered in previous chapters, if improvements do not involve the people who will use them, they are unlikely to meet their needs. Health and social care systems are designed to be person-centred; involving these people in providing guidance and feedback is essential if their perspectives are to be considered effectively. People receiving care have a vested interest in ensuring care is of the best quality, they can contribute important improvement ideas as well as providing very useful viewpoints in response to others. It is always a good plan to involve them as early as possible, in both discussions and decision-making, to allow them to guide you most effectively.

It is also important to remember that stakeholders are not just the people receiving care, those delivering care also need representation, as their views provide additional perspective on the situation. Gathering their views as baseline information before any change is made is important. Measuring what is currently accepted practice will provide you with a 'baseline' to evaluate whether the change being implemented is resulting in improvement. See Chapter 2 for further details of measurement tools and Chapter 6 for the evaluation tools you could use.

As illustrated earlier, in Figure 5.5, a crucial feature of Part 2 of the explanatory MFI is that the PDCA cycles are not only repeated, but that subject to positive evaluation of the previous cycle, they become progressively larger. This means that, as you repeat the PDCA cycles, the focus and context of the testing expands. In practice this may mean, for example, increasing the number of people, or the areas involved in a subsequent cycle. Figure 5.8 highlights a possible approach Elisabeth could adopt.

As Figure 5.8 shows, the repetition of the PDCA cycles, making only one small change from the previous cycle each time, will enable Elisabeth to link the results being achieved with the changes being made. To help you maximise the effectiveness of your planning, Figure 5.9 provides a 'checklist' of tasks to be undertaken and issues to be considered in this stage.

Cycle 1	Cycle 2	Cycle 3	Cycle 4	Cycle 5
Elisabeth delivers handover by using the SBARD tool to structure her handover	Half of the nurses on a day shift deliver handover using the SBARD tool to structure their handover	All of the nurses on a day shift deliver handover using the SBARD tool to structure their handover	All of the nurses on shift over the course of 24 hours deliver handover using the SBARD tool to structure their handover	All of the nurses on shift over a week deliver handover using the SBARD tool to structure their handover

Figure 5.8   Elisabeth's plan for PDCA cycles

Plan

Explain what you want to achieve in an aim statement

Outline the current process and the issues with that process

Recruit team members

Identify possible causes of the 'problem' you want to improve

Identify possible changes or alternatives that might resolve the problem

Consider what might happen when you implement the possible changes, and why

Plan the test of the change, including what data you will collect and how you will collect it

Implement SMART goals

Consider the resources you will need

Establish the actions you need to implement, and the individuals responsible for each

Devise the timeline for the first PDCA cycle - remember PDCA cycles are repeated, so make modifications small

Figure 5.9   Checklist for the elements included in 'Plan' (adapted from Eby, 2021)

While the Plan of PDCA is likely to be the most substantial of the four stages, as it is where the strategy to test an improvement idea is devised, this does not mean the remaining three stages are less important. They are possibly more important, as they are where an idea is subjected to testing, evaluation and refinement.

Activity 5.4   Critical thinking

Preceding chapters and Table 5.1 have introduced you to a range of quality improvement tools and suggested how they could be used to help plan and implement an idea. If you were part of Elisabeth's improvement team, what tools would you suggest she uses during the PDCA stages of the cycles?

Jot down your thoughts in Table 5.5, then review the template answers at the end of the chapter for comparison.

Quality improvement tool name	At which point of the second part of the MFI can it be used?
	Plan
	Do
	Check
	Act

Table 5.5   Quality improvement tools used in Part 2 of the MFI

Do

The 'Do' element of PDCA is where you implement the action plan devised during 'Plan' and keep a written record of the results. A fundamentally important element of this stage is to collect any relevant data, as this will be vital for the next 'Check' stage. There are several tools you can use to capture the data generated in this stage; refer to Chapter 2 for an introduction to measurement and Chapter 6 for more detailed information on evaluation. As Chapter 2 also highlights, it is important to record all problems encountered during this stage, or any unforeseen effects of how you are now working, plus any general observations, as this will add to the information you have to consider during 'Check'.

Check

In 'Check' you are evaluating what has happened and thinking critically to analyse what the results of the change being tested during this PDCA cycle have been. To do this you need to review the aim statement devised in Part 1 of the explanatory MFI and the data gathered in the 'Do' of this cycle to establish:

1. whether your action plan resulted in improvement or not?
2. if there was improvement, was it large or small?
3. whether the improvement you achieved was worth the resources invested in it?

4. what trends are there in the data you collected?

5. whether the new way of working produced any unintended effects, and were these positive or negative?

Elisabeth is likely to find that using a run chart, which was outlined in Chapter 2, is useful at this stage. Run charts are used to record data as it occurs, providing Elisabeth with a visual overview of the changes resulting from each PDCA cycle (Figure 5.9). Elisabeth's run chart is illustrated in Figure 5.10.

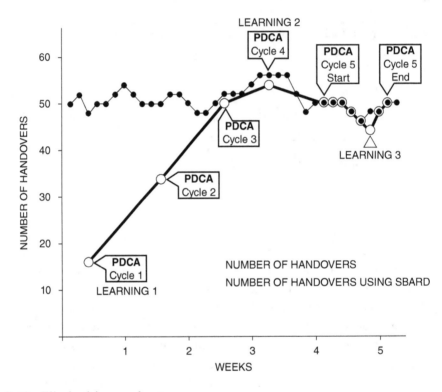

Figure 5.10 Elisabeth's run chart

Figure 5.10 shows the format of handovers over the course of five PDCA cycles. As the number of nurses using the SBARD tool increases it becomes clear that this format is being adopted for most handovers and the two lines on the chart converge.

Elisabeth's run chart, however, provides information on more than just the number of handovers using SBARD. While collecting the **quantitative** data displayed in Figure 5.10, Elisabeth would also be gaining **qualitative** data from those involved. This could be collected in several ways, such as informal individual feedback following use of the SBARD tool and group feedback from ward meeting discussions, for example. Elisabeth could also encourage staff to email her, enabling them to contribute even if they could not attend the other opportunities. The qualitative data collected could further develop Elisabeth's understanding of the change. For example, on Figure 5.10

learning 1, learning 2 and learning 3 are marked; these are points where Elisabeth was helped to understand what happened by the qualitative data.

- Learning 1 identifies Elisabeth's realisation after using SBARD herself that she needed to know the tool; relying upon a 'prompt' sheet made handover less effective.
- Learning 2 indicates where handovers using SBARD were lower in number than anticipated, because a nurse could not find a SBARD prompt sheet, so did not use the tool.
- Learning 3 marks again where handovers using SBARD were less than anticipated, this time because the nurse forgot to use SBARD.

Information like this is of great value to Elisabeth as she checks what has happened, evaluates progress so far and the challenges to be overcome as she plans further PDCA cycles with the team.

Identifying potential unforeseen challenges for quality improvements in practice and strategies for managing these

The most difficult aspect of managing unforeseen challenges is that they are unforeseen because it is hard to plan for something you cannot predict; even the most experienced practitioner may meet an unforeseen challenge when implementing improvement. There are, however, actions that can be undertaken to increase our knowledge and understanding, thus improving our ability to predict the challenges we may face and identify potential solutions. Table 5.6 identifies ten commonly encountered challenges in quality improvement and strategies for managing them.

Challenge	Management strategy
1. **Convincing people that there is a problem**	Use evidence to identify the problem and use relevant patient stories to illustrate the issues.
2. **Convincing people of the solution**	Ensure you have data that supports the solution. Clearly outline the advantages of the change.
3. **Data collection and monitoring**	Make sure you know what data you want to collect at the start and seek support from experts.
4. **Ambitions**	Over-ambitious aims alienate people as they may feel the change is impossible. Match aims and ambitions to what is realistic.
5. **Organisational culture**	Ensure aims match the wider goals of the organisation.
6. **Tribalism and lack of engagement**	Overcoming a perceived lack of ownership and professional boundaries can be difficult. Clarify who owns the problem and solution, agree roles and responsibilities at the start, devise common goals and use shared language.

(Continued)

Table 5.6 (Continued)

Challenge	Management strategy
7. **Leadership**	Effective leadership requires a combination of identifying the new vision while remaining sensitive to the views of others. Aim to be inclusive, use explanation and persuasion.
8. **Motivation**	Relying on staff intrinsic motivation can be effective but enable staff to appreciate that participating in change is a fundamental aspect of their role, not an optional extra.
9. **Sustainability**	Engage everyone in the improvement, as sustainability is unlikely if the improvement is seen as a 'project' or just relies on a few individuals.
10. **Side effects**	Successfully targeting one issue can create problems elsewhere. Be both vigilant about detecting unwanted consequences and willing to learn and adapt.

Table 5.6 Common challenges (adapted from Dixon-Woods et al, 2012)

Act

This is the stage of each PDCA cycle that emphasises the need to develop and apply iterative actions based on evaluation of the preceding cycle. In this stage the focus is on reflecting upon the results of the three previous stages, i.e. 'Plan', 'Do', 'Check'. As shown earlier in Figure 5.5, PDCA cycles are designed to be undertaken repeatedly as it is unlikely you will achieve the improvement aim identified without revising and repeating multiple cycles. At this point you have three possible actions, depending upon what you have learned. From the results of the testing of an improvement idea, you can either:

> *adjust* – modify the change tested in that cycle and repeat the PDCA cycle to learn more; *or*
>
> *abandon* – change your approach entirely. Abandon the idea tested, select a new one, then repeat the PDCA cycle to learn more; *or*
>
> *adopt* – implement the change as routine practice in the area in which it was tested and consider expanding to other areas.

You decide which action to take by returning to the initial three questions of Part 1 of the explanatory MFI. Although we have considered the explanatory MFI in two parts, we must not forget that the two are integrated. After completing each PDCA cycle we must return to Part 1 of the model and reconsider the three initial questions to complete the 'Check' or evaluation element of PDCA. So, by considering whether or not you:

- have achieved what you were trying to accomplish (Question 1);
- have evidence to support that the change is an improvement (Question 2);
- can adapt the change any further to result in greater improvement (Question 3).

the decision to adjust, abandon or adopt is made.

As illustrated in Figure 5.5, in Elisabeth's plan for the PDCA cycles the first cycle tested an improvement idea on a small scale, then in the second, third, fourth and fifth cycles there was a gradual increase in the scale and scope of the testing. PDCA cycles replicate a slowly expanding spiral, with each cycle including just a minor adjustment to the preceding one. Only when evaluation of the data obtained provides conclusive evidence that the improvement has a consistently positive impact has the point been reached when a change should be sustained and embedded within current practice (see Chapter 6 for further details).

Even then, however, thinking about improvement does not stop. Quality improvement is a fundamental everyday activity for nurses and all improvements need to be regularly reviewed, as it may be possible to develop them further. If this is the case, it is time to start applying the explanatory MFI again, testing new ideas to achieve further improvement as part of a continuous improvement culture.

Chapter summary

The delivery of effective and contemporary nursing care depends upon quality improvement, as unless the current state of care provision is constantly reviewed and developed, practice will not advance. The position nurses occupy within any healthcare system places them in a prime position to positively influence and develop care; realising the possibility for improvement and acting to implement new ideas is a fundamental aspect of the role. Successful planning and implementation of improvement requires the application of a diverse range of skills including project monitoring, project management, leadership, data collection and data analysis. These are skills that nursing students of all experience levels either possess or can develop, as they are the same core skills that nurses apply to function effectively in their everyday practice.

Applying a systematic approach to the planning and implementation of an improvement idea increases the chance of its successful adoption in practice. The explanatory MFI is an excellent choice of model, which when combined with other tools and theoretical frameworks provides a useful framework to support nurse-led continuous improvement.

Effective evaluation underpins successful planning and implementation of all improvement ideas. Evaluation must start at the very outset of the planning and implementation stage and remain central throughout the improvement process.

Glossary

Methodology: a specific set of procedures
Qualitative: referring to words
Quantitative: referring to numbers

Answers to activities

Activity 5.2 Communication

Harry only has 30 seconds to outline his idea – so he needs to explain it in a clear and simple fashion. He would need to consider very carefully who the person or people he was talking to were, as this may influence what he says. For example, the language he uses would differ if he was talking to healthcare staff, people who access services, or the general public. Using the prompts identified by Figure 5.3, this is what Harry said when delivering his elevator pitch to the ward manager:

(Prompt 1) 'The change is to alter the ordering of the patient information folders found at each patient's bedside to consistently present the information contained within them in the same order, with each section clearly labelled'.

(Prompt 2) 'The benefit of this change will be that information can be located more quickly. This is important at all times, but especially so in an emergency'.

(Prompt 3) 'I will introduce the change by firstly discussing the idea with staff to gain their support and feedback. I will use the staff views to make sure the plan is as good as it can be. I will then introduce new folders with labelled sections gradually in one of the six bedded bays in the ward. When staff have worked with the new system for one week and provided feedback about what works and what doesn't, the folders will be altered to make them work effectively. We will continue in this way until everyone receiving care on the ward has the new style folders.'

(Prompt 4) 'To achieve this change I need the support of the ward staff.'

(Prompt 5) 'Do you have any questions you would like me to answer?'

Activity 5.3 Critical thinking

These are the tools Harry could use to assist him in applying the first part of the MFI. In the same way as is shown in Table 5.2a by 'stakeholder feedback', it is likely that many of the tools could be useful at more than one stage in the model. You can choose to apply what you think will help you!

Quality improvement tool name	At which point of the first part in the MFI can it be used?
Stakeholder views	
Audit findings	
Complaints	
Friends and Family Test data	
Service user experience feedback	Initial question 1 – 'What are you trying to accomplish?'
Listening to colleagues, people accessing services and carers	
Brain storming	
Reflection upon	
Cost/benefit analysis	

Quality improvement tool name	At which point of the first part in the MFI can it be used?
Stakeholder feedback – staff, people accessing services and the public	Initial question 2 – 'How will you know that the change is an improvement?'
Run charts	
Audit/Re-audit data	
Identify a basket of outcomes and SMART measures	
Literature review	
Stakeholder consultation – including expert opinion	
Process mapping	
Z technique	Initial question 3 – 'What change can you make that will result in improvement?'
Ishikawa	
Affinity/Driver diagram	
Options appraisal	
Business case	

Table 5.2a Quality improvement tools Harry could use in MFI Part 1

Activity 5.4 Critical thinking

These are the tools Elisabeth could use to assist her in applying the second part of the MFI. In the same way as is shown in Table 5.3a by 'stakeholder feedback', it is likely that many of the tools could be helpful at more than one stage in the model. You can choose to apply what you think will help you!

Quality improvement tool name	At which point of the second part of the MFI can it be used?
Gantt chart	Plan
NHS sustainability model	
Stakeholder feedback, analysis and management plan	
Audit data	
Project management	
Logic model	
Stakeholder feedback	Do
Leadership skills and tools	
Stakeholder engagement and management	

(Continued)

Table 5.3a (Continued)

Quality improvement tool name	At which point of the second part of the MFI can it be used?
At this point you will review each of the intended outcomes using the evaluation measures identified at the start. This may involve reapplying tools used in the 'Plan' stage, to review progress.	Check
Gather further stakeholder feedback	
Review the Gantt chart	
Reconsider your application of the NHS sustainability model	
Review stakeholder analysis	
Re-audit data	
Stakeholder feedback	Act
Further application of tools will depend upon whether you decide to adopt, abandon or adapt the learning you have gained from previous stages.	
If you are going to:	
Adopt – consider the NHS sustainability model	
Abandon – go back to Part 1 of the MFI and start over	
Adapt – go back to Part 1 of the MFI, decide what modification to the previous change is needed and implement it in the next PDCA cycle	

Table 5.3a   Quality improvement tools used in Part 2 of the MFI

Further reading

Lee, CS, Larson, DB (2014) Beginner's guide to practice quality improvement using the Model for Improvement. *Journal of the American College of Radiology*, 11 (12): 1131–1136.

Article focusing on the application of the MFI.

Useful websites

http://www.ihi.org/resources/Pages/HowtoImprove/default.aspx Institute for Healthcare Improvement (IHI) – How to improve. Excellent site that uses the Model for Improvement and a range of eye-catching formats to guide improvement work.

http://squire-statement.org/index.cfm?fuseaction=Page.ViewPage&PageID=471 SQUIRE 2.0

Chapter 6 · Evaluating and sustaining improvement

Michelle Croston and Daniel Heggie

NMC Future Nurse: Standards of Proficiency for Registered Nurses

This chapter will address the following platforms and proficiencies:

Platform 5: Leading and managing care and working in teams

5.12 understand the mechanisms that can be used to influence organisational change and public policy, demonstrating the development of political awareness and skills.

Platform 6: Improving safety and quality of care

6.4 demonstrate an understanding of the principles of improvement methodologies, participate in all stages of audit activity and identify appropriate quality improvement strategies.

6.7 understand how the quality and effectiveness of nursing care can be evaluated in practice, and demonstrate how to use service delivery evaluation and audit findings to bring about continuous improvement.

Platform 7: Co-ordinating care

7.12 demonstrate an understanding of the processes involved in developing a basic business case for additional care funding by applying knowledge of finance, resources and safe staffing levels.

I've done all this work to try and make things better, how can I be sure it is actually better?

(Louise, registered nurse learning disability)

I don't see the point in all this effort to improve, new things never last long anyway.

(Ari, 3rd year mental health field nursing student)

Introduction

As both Ari and Louise have highlighted above, quality improvement is often seen as complex and difficult to evaluate, spread and sustain within a busy clinical environment. Hopefully, by now, as you have worked through and completed the activities in this book, you are starting to see the fog lift and feel invigorated and more confident about your contribution to improving services. As you will now understand, each chapter in this book builds on previous ones and connects to those following; this reflects the complex, integrated journey of undertaking successful improvement, much like a game of snakes and ladders.

This chapter will enable you to use what you've learned to this point, while introducing key concepts and tools you can use to help you evaluate, spread and effectively sustain a quality improvement. Although it may feel counterintuitive, it is important to invest time at the start of any improvement to consider these issues. This chapter will therefore focus on identifying appropriate ways to evaluate your improvement, suggest ways in which you can develop a robust dissemination strategy and sustain the change for the future.

The history of improvement and change in healthcare

Since its inception in 1948, the NHS has been involved in continuous improvement and change, which is also evident in other health and social care settings.

This has been essential as the NHS and other health and social care providers have been required to meet the ever-changing demands alongside continuing pressure to provide a high-quality service, for an increasing population with limited financial resources. As highlighted in previous chapters, this has required all healthcare professionals to be innovative in what they do. However, without learning from what does not work well or ensuring any effective improvement activity is sustainable, positive change will be limited at best and opportunities missed to recognise and celebrate success. As mentioned in Chapter 4, without adequate sustainability planning, an improvement is 70% more likely to fail (NHS Institute for Innovation and Improvement, 2010); therefore, developing the core skills to critically evaluate and sustain an improvement through engaging with this chapter means your improvement efforts are more likely to be successful and you are unlikely to end up feeling like Louise and Ari who we heard from at the start of the chapter.

Evaluating an improvement

Before we go any further with considering 'evaluation' it is important to understand what we mean by this term in the context of quality improvement. The NHS Institute for Innovation and Improvement (2005) suggest evaluation is the systematic assessment of the implementation and impact of a project, programme or initiative. The purpose of the evaluation is to help judge the value of a project by gathering information about it in a structured way for the purpose of making better informed decisions. Evaluations are also of benefit not only to the project team but to others who are considering making similar changes. Evaluation enables others to learn from your experiences. Evaluations help us to share the key learning from the project and identify what worked well and what was difficult to implement into clinical practice. If project results are communicated in the right way, they can be used to inform new policies, new ways of working and future research.

As was introduced in Chapter 2, it is important to consider how you will evaluate your project to help yourself and others to understand which methods and innovations work to improve quality. It is important to consider from the start what you intend to evaluate and how to do this. At the start of any improvement, it is important to be **pragmatic** regarding how much change is possible within the boundaries of the improvement initiative as this will help to guide the evaluation. Please refer to Chapter 4 for how to create effective aims. Having clear aims is crucial for helping clarify what is being evaluated, as is highlighted in Figure 6.1, which outlines best practice in evaluating improvement.

1. Take a collaborative approach to agreeing a clear theory of change.
2. Plan for evaluation at the beginning.
3. Be clear about your purpose and design evaluation with key audiences in mind.
4. Think about evaluation when setting improvement targets – identify and separate out stretch and evaluative goals.
5. Adopt a formative learning approach to evaluation and align evaluation design to programme design.
6. Be flexible and plan for change, review your evaluation model regularly.
7. Build in ongoing evaluation throughout improvement projects and use data to inform quality improvement plans.

Figure 6.1 Best practice in evaluating healthcare improvement projects (The Health Foundation 2011, p10)

It can be difficult to evaluate an improvement initiative if you are unclear what theory of change you will use, so this is an early consideration; Chapter 3 explores change theory and Table 5.1 in Chapter 5 considers how theories relate to each other, so revisit these sections if you need a refresher. Table 6.1 is a quick reference guide to where evaluation and dissemination is explored within each of the change models discussed in Chapter 3. Please refer to the one you are using and familiarise yourself with the evaluation sections of it in more depth. Table 6.1 provides an example of how the evaluation elements from the different models for improvement have been used to assist with the evaluation of a quality improvement initiative.

Being clear about how change will be achieved will help to ensure the correct data is collected to enable successful evaluation of the improvement. Evaluation provides a check that (1) you are doing things right and (2) that you are also doing the right thing.

Evaluating efforts to improve quality improvement can be challenging and complex due to multiple different stakeholders who need data and who will be looking for slightly different things when assessing how effective a project has been (Davidoff and Batalden, 2005). For example, funders may want to see the economic benefits, managers may be interested in how the resources have been better used and healthcare professionals may focus more on the benefits to the person accessing care. When considering the dissemination strategy, it is also very important to consider feedback to the service user group as they are key stakeholders in any improvement initiative. Ensuring you communicate effectively with stakeholders is key for ensuring any

Model	Where in the model evaluation is explored	Practice-based example
Six stage project management guide (2010)	Sustain and share is the section of the model that explores how you will know change has been successful and how you will ensure that new ways of working are sustained.	Joanne had successfully developed a project within her community team that ensured National Early Warning Score (NEWS2) scores were completed during the first home visit, something that was often overlooked. Joanne shared her project at a regional team meeting, which resulted in another team implementing the idea for their community team.
NHS Change Model (2012)	Spread and adoption	Joanne is invited to a national meeting to discuss her work. After the meeting a member of another community team approaches her to see how they could develop this within their team.
Kotter 8 Steps	Step 7: Build the change and make it stick	Joanne is worried that as she has been promoted and won't be in the team the project won't carry on without her. Joanne discusses her concerns with her manager, who explores ways to ensure that the practice is now adopted as a normal standard of practice within the team. Joanne's manager agrees to build in an audit of NEWS scores at first visit to the overall service audit plan.
Lewin	Refreeze	Joanne makes this the new normal as the team are now routinely using the NEWS2 as part of their initial assessment of patients. When a new member of staff joins the team, this process is discussed with them as being standard practice within the team and is therefore embedded within the local induction programme.
The model for improvement	C – check what has happened A – Act on what is learnt	Joanne helps the team to see what they have learnt by undertaking the project and clearly demonstrates the impact on patient outcomes. As a result, the team start exploring other projects that they could develop using the lessons they have learnt.

Table 6.1 Examples of change models and their application in evaluation

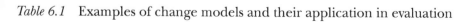

improvement is sustainable. However, it is important that the messages are adapted for different audiences, taking into consideration that different stakeholders have different priorities and communication preferences. You will therefore need to identify the target audience(s), then creatively design a dissemination strategy tailored for each one to ensure the improvement has the greatest possible impact. Complete Activity 6.1 now to help you do this.

Activity 6.1   Communication

1. Consider how you might communicate with the different stakeholders associated with your improvement idea.
2. Think about how you will create regular feedback loops for yourself as you progress the improvement.

Completing Table 6.2 will help you to consider how to effectively communicate with different stakeholders – being as specific as you can, produce a plan to address the needs of each stakeholder group involved in your improvement.

Stakeholders	What are they interested in within the project?	What is the best way to communicate this with the stakeholders?	In what time frame should I communicate this information?
Manager			
Project funders			
People using the service			

Table 6.2   Effective Communication Techniques

Once you have completed this activity, compare your answers with the worked example at the end of the chapter.

Having considered your stakeholders along with how and what to communicate with them, Activity 6.2 is designed to help you think about the steps involved in creating an evaluation strategy.

Activity 6.2   Measuring

You are a member of the project team helping Elisabeth to evaluate her improvement. Refer to Elisabeth's story at the start of Part 2 of the book, review Table 4.1 and read the information in Chapter 4 discussing how the SMART aim for her improvement idea was outlined. Then devise an appropriate evaluation strategy for Elisabeth to use.

Questions to consider:

1. What data (information) you want to collect – qualitative, quantitative or both?
2. Is there a comparative group?
3. Will before measures (baseline measures) and after measure be taken?
4. Will feedback be gathered? If so when and from whom?
5. Will you need to use a combination of measures?

Discuss your responses to questions 1–5 and outline evaluation with your lecturer or someone in your practice area; this could be a peer, a colleague experienced in QI or someone in the research and innovation department.

A logic model can be a useful evaluation tool to use. This is a graphic depiction (road map) that presents the relationships between resources, activities, outputs, outcomes and impact of the project. It depicts the relationship between the improvement activities and their intended effects (Wyatt Knowlton and Phillips, 2013).

There are several versions and interpretations of the logic model concept. Perigo and Callaghan (2011) adapted the logic model to make it more clinically relevant and to support commissioners and providers of healthcare to focus on health outcomes to support the evaluation of improvement initiatives. Their adaptation provides clinical and commissioning clarity on:

Step 1 – Who you should be caring for

Step 2 – What the evidence base and quality interventions are and who should be involved

Step 3 – Evidence that the intervention(s) have taken place (consider established audit criteria)

Step 4 – An understanding of how to measure the intervention and what it means (outcome)

Step 5 – An understanding of the long-term effects of the intervention.

When considering how to best use a logic model in the evaluation stage of an improvement initiative it is useful to focus on steps 3, 4 and 5 as steps 1 and 2 should already have been clarified when justifying the change and its scope (see Chapter 4 for further information on these topics); these will now be discussed further to aid your understanding of how these steps may be used in your evaluation.

Step 3: Evidence that the intervention(s) have taken place (consider established audit criteria*):* This can be achieved by developing a set of criteria that you will revisit once the improvement initiative is complete, to ensure these have been met.

Step 4: An understanding of how to measure the intervention and what it means (outcome): It is important to establish what you are measuring at the start of the improvement initiative as this enables you to evaluate whether there have been any changes and to what extent these may be related to the improvement itself.

Step 5: An understanding of the long-term effects of the intervention: At the start of the improvement it may be hard to consider what the longer-term effects may be; these may evolve as the project does. However, the long-term effects of the improvement are important to consider in any evaluation and engaging with the broadest range of perspectives by engaging with the key stakeholders will help to identify the potential long-term effects.

The benefits of using the logic model are that it can help staff easily develop and lead improvement initiatives, while ensuring any patient safety issues can be identified and measured before potential adverse effects occur. The model enables and guides the user towards measuring what matters and helps you to understand the outcomes of the intervention. Using this tool also helps you to create a framework for appropriate indicators to support the **audit cycle**, providing a mechanism for continuous quality improvement through ongoing evaluation of the change.

When evaluation is not done well, it can have a negative impact on several different levels. For example, it can render an improvement as wasted effort or can mean that the project is viewed as lacking in credibility, both of which can impact on efforts to improve patient care. Several different types of evaluation exist, but the most common are summative and formative (The Health Foundation, 2015). Summative evaluations provide an overall overview of the entire project and are normally performed at the end when all the data is available to enable the team to assess whether the intervention has been a success against the stated goals. Formative evaluations are usually used at various stages of project implementation and can provide vital information on how best to revise and modify the work taking place. Formative evaluation can help to establish not only whether the improvement goals are being met, but also how and why they are being met within that particular environment. It is likely that both summative and formative evaluation will be needed to ensure comprehensive evaluation against the original objective or improvement goal as this can provide crucial learning for future initiatives. As a student you will be very familiar with the terms formative and summative assessment in relation to academic assignments; formative assignments being those designed to assess ongoing learning to help you identify strengths and weaknesses in your work to enable you to develop. Summative assessments, on the other hand, are those you submit for formal marking and grading at the end of a period of learning; this feedback can only be used to enhance future work. You can think of summative and formative evaluations in quality improvement as undertaking the same roles.

Building in sustainability

Chapter 4 considered the place sustainability has in helping to scope an improvement idea and particularly to ensure the development of SMART objectives. Table 4.1, which focused on what SMART aims for Elisabeth's improvement idea might look like, illustrated this. In Chapter 4 sustainability was referred to as being achieved when a new way of working becomes 'business as usual'. However, sustainability is still a step in the quality improvement process that is often brushed to one side as something to 'think about later'. It can be easy to rush past this step in the excitement of realising the potential for the change to result in what you perceive to be a better service, process or service user/staff outcome. After all, why wouldn't an amazingly innovative project be sustained automatically? Unfortunately, unless sustainability is built in from the start even the best improvements are, as we learned earlier, almost three times more likely to fail than succeed. Here, we build on what you already know about evaluation and sustainability. Solid planning and preparation is required to maximise the long-term impact of an improvement.

Take a moment to think about a time when you tried something new – this could be a new hobby, hairstyle or way of doing things at work – and complete Activity 6.3 to help you start thinking about how to sustain change.

Activity 6.3   Critical thinking

- How long did this change last?
- What made this change easier?
- What made it harder to keep up?
- What might have helped you to keep going or persevere with this new 'thing'?

Jot down your responses, then compare them with the sample answer at the end of the chapter, then use these responses when completing Activity 6.4.

As you have realised by now, without adequate preparation even the best quality improvement idea will barely make a splash in the huge ocean of change. This can be known as the improvement evaporation effect or initiative decay (NHS Institute for Innovation and Improvement, 2010). Understanding your short- and long-term goals and keeping them SMART, as discussed earlier, will help you avoid this. In addition, being clear about the value of the proposed improvement will help you convince others, particularly if conflict arises.

It might seem unnecessary to consider conflict when you have such an exciting or obvious quality improvement idea, but having considered that sustainable change might not be appreciated by everyone so applying the transferable empathy skills you are developing during your wider studies offers you a unique opportunity to 'Find Value for Everyone' (NHS Institute for Innovation and Improvement, 2010; Mortimer et al, 2018).

Finding value

Mortimer et al (2018) discuss the need to consider sustainability a cornerstone of healthcare. An improvement must enhance patient outcomes and show sustainability and affordability to ensure it is high in value, worth the effort and time. Since conception, a characteristic of healthcare has been that it is in a constant cycle of change and continuous improvement. Healthcare should be considered not only in terms of what can be delivered to an individual today but building in effective sustainability could mean an improvement could also have an impact on a wider, future population (Atkinson et al, 2010).

Most sustainability will be considered at the very beginning of your project, such as when writing a business case. To find more information on a business case please refer to Chapter 4. Writing an ironclad business case involves answering the key questions that form part of Part 1 of the MFI:

1. What are we trying to accomplish?
2. How will we know change is an improvement?
3. What changes can we make that will result in improvement?

This ensures you understand your objectives and goals and helps gain buy-in for a project from key stakeholders, along with financial resource where necessary. Essentially, to help get others on board with what you or others want to do, everyone needs to understand the why, which will also minimise and mitigate potential conflict.

These three key questions are essential to help you know what you want to achieve, by focusing on identifying the value and impact of any improvement idea. The PDCA cycle is not perfect; however, the failure of the PDCA can often be attributed to human error, misunderstanding or lack of preparation (Reed & Card, 2015). As discussed in Chapter 4 and here, effectively measuring improvement or evaluating and then sustaining the change is significantly hindered if you do not know what you set out to achieve.

Knowing what you want to achieve and the impact it can make is key for sustainability, as even with the best laid plans improvement can be unpredictable and the results you expect may not be what happens. Running a small-scale improvement more effectively, therefore, enables long-term implementation. Implementing multiple PDCA cycles, using appropriate evaluation criteria, enables continuous learning and demonstration of effect, measuring whether your need for improvement is reasonable and, if so, how to improve your initiative for an additional, potentially larger-scale improvement (NHS England, 2021).

Activity 6.4 will help you to understand how you can effectively evaluate and sustain an improvement activity.

Activity 6.4   Reflection

You may know the proposed change is one that will give continued benefits, improve services and have the ability to evolve into even better things, but have you considered that sustaining a change may not always be viewed positively by others?

Using either an improvement idea of your own, or Elisabeth's as an example:

- How do you think you or Elisabeth may overcome negative attitudes toward the proposed change?
- What actions could you or Elisabeth take to help others see the benefits?

Jot down your responses and discuss with your peers, practice supervisor or lecturer. Consider how this might apply to your own improvement idea.

NHS Sustainability Model and readiness for change

Chapter 4 explored how the NHS Sustainability Model can be used as a diagnostic tool to assess key considerations for sustaining an improvement. A reminder of these elements or branches comprising this model can be found in Table 6.3.

Process	Staff	Organisation
Benefits beyond helping patients	Training and involvement	Fit with goals and culture
Credibility of benefits	Behaviours	Infrastructure
Adaptability	Senior leaders	
Monitoring progress	Clinical leaders	

Table 6.3   NHS Sustainability Model (2017): key branches

This model identifies three key branches to be considered: process, staff and organisation. You will find an explanation of each branch in Chapter 4. As explained there, these branches allow us to consider various aspects of the context within which a proposed change will take place; from the people to the culture and credibility of the improvement idea you are proposing and why. However, knowing about these branches alone cannot ensure sustainability; here we illustrate how they can be applied by considering them in terms of the readiness for change. Effective application of the branches requires adoption of four key values: (a) be for people; (b) be fair; (c) be resilient; and (d) be efficient (Moldovan, 2020).

Adopting and combining these values with the NHS Sustainability Model can result in a value-based sustainability framework as shown in Table 6.4.

	Corresponding parts		
Readiness values	**Resilient and efficient**	**Be fair**	**Be for the people**
NHS Sustainability Model	**Process**	**Staff**	**Organisation**
	Benefits beyond helping patients	Training and involvement	Fit with goals and culture
	Credibility of benefits	Behaviours	Infrastructure
	Adaptability	Senior leaders	
	Monitoring progress	Clinical leaders	

Table 6.4   Readiness values combined with the NHS Sustainability Model

However, motivation to change will be the greatest influence on the success or failure of any quality improvement. Moldovan (2020) explains that lack of motivation is often driven by the lack of evidence and data; for example, often resistance is caused by not knowing 'X causes Y issue and Z is the resolution' (Auerbach et al, 2007; NHS Institute for Innovation and Improvement, 2010). Completing Activity 6.5 provides an opportunity for you to consider the readiness values and sustainability branches outlined in Table 6.4 in relation to the area where you want to implement change, to see how the proposed improvement fits and what work you will need to do before beginning.

Activity 6.5   Building knowledge

This activity provides an opportunity to consider the NHS Sustainability Model and the Readiness Values (Table 6.4) to help determine what steps you need to complete before starting an improvement. Use the NHS Sustainability Model resources information in Chapter 4 if needed.

Don't forget: frequently evaluating how things will work will only serve you well, i.e., your future self will thank you for doing this preparatory work at the start.

Using your personal skills to support sustained improvement in practice

Whether you think it is true or not, you are shaping up to become a health and social care leader. Your leadership style will have a huge effect on the sustainability of your quality improvement efforts (Sfantou et al, 2017). As discussed in Chapter 2, the leadership qualities and skills you deploy when leading an improvement can make the difference between success and failure. Box 6.1 summarises some examples of leadership theories, each likely to have a different impact on how sustainable an improvement is if used to guide its development and implementation.

Box 6.1   Some leadership theories

- Compassionate
- Transformational
- Transactional
- Autocratic
- Collective
- Laissez-faire
- Task-oriented
- Relationship-oriented leadership

If you haven't already investigated leadership styles and how they relate to sustaining effective improvement, go back to Chapters 2 and 3 to refresh your memory before completing Activity 6.6.

Activity 6.6   Leadership

Consider which of these styles will help implement your now sustainable quality improvement and why or in what way? When you have finished compare your responses with the worked example at the end of this chapter and talk to the staff teaching the leadership elements of your course or leaders where you work.

Disseminating improvement

After an improvement initiative is complete, and as a project is progressing, if you want to share interim findings, it is important to consider how to present and showcase the findings. The quality improvement community and wider stakeholders must understand what improvements can be replicated to bring about improvement on a larger scale. Sharing and disseminating learning therefore helps to build and develop the improvement knowledge base.

When considering how to disseminate findings it is worth bearing in mind that a well-designed dissemination strategy can improve access to your work and in doing so increase the chances of it being used much more broadly to improve patient outcomes, inform clinical guidelines and transform clinical practice (Grimshaw et al, 2006; Flodgren et al, 2016; Murad, 2017). To ensure this happens, a dissemination strategy needs to be carefully planned and consideration given to the types of messages you want to get across and the best way to communicate these to various audiences or consumers of the knowledge you wish to share (Wilson et al, 2010; Tabak et al, 2012).

Considering who will be interested in the improvement and who the target audience(s) are is crucial. During this phase of the process, it is worth considering the political context and any implications of the project for the organisation, and key stakeholders, including possible counter issues that need to be addressed during dissemination. Activity 6.7 is designed to help you start developing this plan.

Activity 6.7   Communication

Consider the following: who is the audience(s) and what is the best way to share the results with this group of people?

Once you've jotted down your ideas, speak to someone in each target group for their views on how effective the ideas you have identified might be for them.

There are many ways to disseminate improvement findings. It is important to consider how to disseminate your findings locally to the team who have been involved and supported the improvement process; a stage that can often get overlooked.

As illustrated in Chapter 5, the SQUIRE guidelines (Ogrinc et al, 2016) provide a framework for reporting new knowledge about interventions that are designed to improve healthcare; many professional and academic journals will not consider improvement project reports for publication if they do not adhere to these guidelines. You may be encouraged as part of your formal programme of study to use the SQUIRE structure when reporting an improvement project for assessment as they are designed to support best practice in QI reporting. Using these guidelines as a template can help you provide a systematic and comprehensive record of the improvement process and key findings for dissemination. It may not be appropriate to use every section of the SQUIRE guideline in every case, so be prepared to adapt it to suit what is appropriate for the particular project or situation (Ogrinc et al, 2016).

Professional conferences are a good way to share information with a wider audience (see the below case study). Consider which conferences would have the greatest impact in terms of your target audience(s) and what messages you want to deliver based on the type of delegate/attendee before pursuing this.

Case study   Presenting at a conference

Jake's line manager asked him to consider presenting his improvement project findings at an upcoming conference. Initially, Jake declined and suggested that he thought his manager may be better placed to present the findings on behalf of the team. However, the line manager offered to support Jake to develop the presentation and provided him with opportunities to practice his presentation prior to the conference. As the date of the conference approached, Jake's line manager met with him to identify any support that he might need. After the conference Jake reflected on his experience and remarked that he was grateful to have been given the opportunity to move out of his comfort zone to present the project and for the support and encouragement he had had from the team. He used this experience as the focus for a reflective piece for inclusion in his practice portfolio.

You may wish to publish your findings in a scientific journal so that they reach a larger target audience. If you decide to publish, you should seek guidance from your lecturer, mentor or other colleagues unless you have published before – this will save you a lot of wasted time and effort in choosing the most appropriate journal and requirements, regarding publication fees for example (See the below case study).

Case study   Submitting an article to a peer reviewed journal

Jacinta was delighted to receive excellent feedback on her quality improvement project that she had submitted as part of her course. She read the comments to look for suggestions on how she may improve her work for next time, when she noticed that one of her lecturers had suggested she consider converting this assessed work into a manuscript for submission for publication in a peer reviewed professional journal. Unsure what to do, Jacinta made an appointment to speak with the lecturer who had made the comments. During this meeting Jacinta received some invaluable advice, i.e. to decide which journal would be best suited to publish her work. You can do this by reading the scope on the journal website re: topic areas, readership type, types of articles accepted. Once she had established which journal to target, she downloaded the author guidelines for the journal website. As this was a new experience for Jacinta, her lecturer offered to support her with the process.

You should also present to the relevant service user and public groups that may have an interest in or be affected by your findings. If you involved these stakeholders in the improvement work throughout they will be key partners in all dissemination activity, which will help maximise success. The type of report required for this purpose is often referred to as a lay summary and consists of a summary of the main findings that is designed for a non-specialist audience. The lay summary should use plain English, no jargon and if required, explain any technical terms that have been used. See the resources section at the end of this chapter for a useful link to a guide on how to write a lay summary; ideally, you should encourage any people using services or members of the public engaged with the project to help create this.

Social media is another good way to share your findings with a variety of different groups. If you choose to use this method, you will need to consider which platform is:

- most appropriate for the information you want to communicate;
- most likely to be used by your target audience; and
- what you would like the recipients to do with that information (call to action).

By virtue of its design, social media elicits quick responses and enables the creation of a rapid dialogue between you and the audience, so careful planning on when to release posts, for example, is necessary to ensure you build in time to monitor responses and respond when necessary (Sloan and Quan-Haase, 2017). It is also very important to know which platform is most prevalent to which group you are targeting, understanding that platforms can become obsolete very quickly. When communicating on social media, you must adhere to your code of professional conduct (NMC, 2018a) and professional body social media guidelines (NMC, 2015) and seek advice locally from your lecturer or practice supervisor.

There may also be other forums or discussion boards you could consider, including those led by service users or the general public. Spend some time to explore what options might be open to you when developing the project dissemination strategy and review the below case study.

Case study   Involving service users in improvement

Elisabeth continued to pursue improving handover practice. She now focused on improving bedside handovers and was in the very early stages of planning what to do. She had noticed that during the bedside handover process, jargon, abbreviations and acronyms were often used. This made her feel she wanted to stay behind to describe in lay terms to the person accessing care what had been discussed.

She decided to seek feedback on the experiences of bedside handover from service users and carers in her area. Hearing their stories helped Elisabeth understand how they were able to grasp what was happening, while also noting how difficult this was and how overwhelmed the process made them feel. She therefore identified individuals from a local service user and carer group to join the project team, ensuring their perspectives informed every aspect of the subsequent improvement process to enhance bedside handover.

Chapter summary

This chapter has explored how to evaluate, sustain and effectively disseminate the findings from quality improvement in practice.

Using the tools and activities provided here should ensure your improvement effort is as successful as possible. Investing time at the start to build in evaluation and sustainability will markedly increase the chance of success and your ability to lead impactful change in practice. From now on, do consider how you can use what you have learned about identifying strategies to sustain, knowing your leadership style, identifying appropriate ways to evaluate and how you might disseminate your project; although we highly encourage it, shouting from the roof tops will only get you so far.

Glossary

Pragmatic: dealing with things sensibly and realistically in a way that is based on practical rather than theoretical considerations.

Audit cycle: the process that auditors use; involves five steps – preparation, criteria selection, measuring, making and maintaining improvements.

Audit criteria: the standard you evaluate the subject matter against. Without a firm audit criterion, it is harder to make clear recommendations for how to improve what has been audited.

Answers to activities

Activity 6.1 Communication

Stakeholders	What are they interested in within the project?	What is the best way to communicate this with the stakeholders?	In what time frame should I communicate this information
Manager	Is this a good use of staff time and resources	Regular update meetings, creating a progress report template to help	Throughout the project at regular time frames 4–6 weekly
Project funders	Is this work good value for money? What are the project outcomes?	Formal report and meeting with presentation	At the end of the project
Patient groups	How will this improve my care?	Service user leaflet and poster in the waiting room	At the start and the end of the project

Activity 6.3 Critical thinking

Whenever I get a new haircut, I am never happy with it for the first couple of days. It's harder to know why I had my hair cut, it feels strange, my head is a little lighter, maybe a bit colder.

However, this is made easier by the compliments and good feedback I get from people. This really helped me get through this. Finally, as it starts to grow a little, I can really see the benefit and can appreciate the work that went into my haircut.

Activity 6.4 Reflection

Elisabeth would need to establish her 'Why?' as seen in Chapter 4. She can do this by looking at the structure of the place where she intends to improve, the process, staff and organisation. Combined with the readiness values, by understanding the people, being effective and resilient she will be prepared for any bump in the road or predict any conflict she might face.

Activity 6.5 Building knowledge

Having looked at all the models, it would be best for you to begin by looking at where you are trying to improve. Does it have a dedicated improvement team, or a dedicated individual? These people will be a great source of information and may already have completed a relevant readiness review. If not, you have the readiness review from this book (this chapter and Chapter 4) to help you.

Activity 6.6 Leadership

How leadership theory may support sustainability

- *Compassionate*: Compassionate leadership is a powerful facilitator at each stage of the problem-solving process. Staff are more likely to engage with innovation if they feel listened to, valued and supported as this provides a sense of psychological safety.
- *Transformational*: Transformational leaders can inspire others, inspire people to do what is needed. This can help overcome conflict, help with sustainability and morale.
- *Transactional*: Transactional leaders are very task based. As you will know by now, improvement is an ever-changing process. So, having some organisational skills that help keep you on track is a necessity.
- *Collective*: Collective leaders apply leadership to all, find those people who flourish at certain tasks, despite their level with an organisation. Each member has their own value.
- *Laissez-faire*: Being able to take a step back is just as important as being hands on. It can often be counterproductive to be constantly waiting around or asking lots of questions; although you want to avoid team members getting the impression you are not interested or do not care.
- *Relationship-oriented*: Building relationships can be the make or break of a sustainable improvement. You will need to find the key influencers, wherever and whoever they are, to help engage others with new ways of working.

Arguably all leadership theory can be used to help progress improvement and building in the sustainability required. Knowing the advantages and disadvantages of each, plus where your strengths and weaknesses lie (as considered in Chapter 2 and will be revisited in Chapter 8), will serve you well.

Useful websites

https://youtu.be/HY8AWSkKRWQ Logic models – A 2.48 minute video providing more information on logic models.

https://www.betterevaluation.org Better Evaluation website – Examples of what to consider in respect of your approach to evaluating a quality improvement initiative.

https://bit.ly/3Oyoj4F In a nutshell: how to write a lay summary – Guidance for writing a lay summary of a quality improvement initiative.

Part 3

Moving forward: introducing Florence

Catherine Delves-Yates and Gillian Janes

This third part of the textbook will enable you to understand the potential for quality improvement to develop over the foreseeable future and the opportunities this will bring for nursing and the delivery of services. Again, in a similar way to the previous parts of the book, we will also help you to understand the terminology used and, most importantly, continue to recognise how quality improvement can become a feature of our everyday practice.

At the start of each chapter you will hear from a number of registered nurses and nursing students, who are very likely to be sharing the challenges and asking the questions you are as you work upon developing your quality improvement skills.

Before you start to read the chapters in this part, however, we would like to introduce you to Florence Kidogo, who is going to share her thoughts on how she can develop her quality improvement skills as she starts her career as a registered nurse. As we progress through this part of the book we will refer back to Florence and identify both strategies and opportunities she may not have considered.

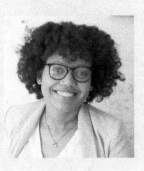

Greetings! My name is Florence Kidogo. I am 28 and in two months' time I will have completed my nursing programme. Yeah! So exciting, but a bit scary too. For me this is such an achievement, and it is something I have wanted for a very long time. Before I started the nursing programme I worked part-time as a Health Care Assistant (HCA), mainly on night shifts. I knew I wanted to be a registered nurse when I was a teenager, but I also knew that, for me, it was better to wait until my two children were at school. As soon as this was the case I had the time to go to university.

I really enjoyed all of the nursing programme, even though I had to work hard to manage all of the studying. I loved the placements too, but enjoyed being in the community the best. Looking after patients in their own homes is, I think, how we should care for so many patients, especially those with long-term illnesses. When you are sick you want to be at home!

(Continued)

(Continued)

Over this final year of the programme it has seemed as if 'everything just came together' and I really enjoyed that in the theory we developed a plan for a quality improvement. My improvement focused upon an aspect of care for patients being nursed in the community – which is where I am hoping I will be able to work as a Staff Nurse.

In fact, next week I have an interview for a Band 5 community Staff Nurse post. This really is my dream job, so I have been thinking very carefully about what I can bring to the post. I know that I still have a great deal to learn, but I think that what I learnt from my nursing programme, in particular the final year, is going to be a solid foundation. I have been reading the job description for the community Staff Nurse post, and I was really pleased to see it mention that I am expected to have 'an active role in quality improvement activities, working in partnership with stakeholders'. I really like the fact that, as part of my nursing role, if something I do with the patients doesn't seem to work well, or doesn't give the best patient experience, I can work on a way to improve it. Yeah! That seems to be so very sensible to me, especially as, according to the job description, I could do this together with the patients and other staff members. I think that working in this way would result in an improvement, not only for the patients, but for the other staff too. It just seems to be common sense to me that if the staff are involved in devising an improvement plan and then carrying it out, there is much more chance of everyone being happy and following the plan. When I was an HCA, before my nursing programme, I worked with a Charge Nurse who was truly excellent in getting everyone to work together. If anything didn't work as well as it could do, she would always say, 'what can we do to make this work better?' I think that is a really good question and something that, as a nurse, I can also do.

I have decided that I am going to make sure that I take the work I did for my improvement project with me, which is really relevant to the care delivered by the community nursing team. I know that I still have lots to learn, and I will tell the interview panel that, but I am good at listening to patients, to see what they think can be better. That is how I got the idea for the improvement plan I devised during my nursing degree. They might be interested in seeing if my improvement would provide better care for their patients too.

So, fingers crossed – and arms and legs and eyes as my children always say!! Here's hoping that the interview goes well and that I can not only start my nursing career as a community Staff Nurse, but that I get the opportunity to implement my improvement plan in real life.

That would be so perfect!

Chapter 7 · Quality improvement

The next decade

Gillian Janes and Catherine Delves-Yates

NMC Future Nurse: Standards of Proficiency for Registered Nurses

This chapter will address the following platforms and proficiencies:

Platform 1: Being an accountable professional

1.19 act as an ambassador, upholding the reputation of their profession and promoting public confidence in nursing, health and care services.

Platform 5: Leading and managing care and working in teams

5.12 understand the mechanisms that can be used to influence organisational change and public policy, demonstrating the development of political awareness and skills.

Platform 6: Improving safety and quality of care

6.6 identify the need to make improvements and proactively respond to potential hazards that may affect the safety of people.

Platform 7: Co-ordinating care

7.13 demonstrate an understanding of the importance of exercising political awareness throughout their career, to maximise the influence and effect of registered nursing on quality of care, patient safety and cost effectiveness.

Chapter aims

After reading this chapter you should be able to:

- critique current progress in improving the quality of healthcare;
- identify future priorities for quality improvement as a developing discipline;
- explore the potential for nurses and nursing in quality improvement within the context of a multidisciplinary team.

I've surprised myself with how many ideas for improvement I can generate. I was even OK last week sharing an idea with other nurses and members of the multidisciplinary team, but I was a bit shocked when my assessor asked what the service users and families thought of the idea – and how I planned to involve them in it!

(Ed, 3rd year student)

I'm definitely more confident about the fundamentals of quality improvement but working out what needs ethical approval is still confusing. My everyday nursing practice is based on ethical principles and upholds the NMC Code – so my practice is governed by more than the agreement of an ethics committee but working out whether I need and how to get approval to talk to or involve colleagues, when what we are doing is part of our everyday reflection on practice and attempts to improve care, isn't always straightforward.

(Raj, 2nd year student)

Introduction

Previous chapters have considered the relevance of quality improvement for nurses and guided you through the process of identifying and leading an improvement in practice. This chapter focuses on current progress in building the evidence base for quality improvement, improvement practice and the future priorities for the discipline, to enable you to consider what contribution both the profession as a whole and you as an individual can offer. As Ed highlights at the start of the chapter, nurses frequently identify areas where improvement is required, but as Raj's experience illustrates, even when you understand the principles of quality improvement, translating this to practice is not easy.

Where are we now?

Quality improvement has a very long history, stretching back to Florence Nightingale and the 1800s (Sheingold and Hahn, 2014). Over the last 30 years, healthcare organisations have been encouraged to adopt a continuous improvement approach, including building QI capability in the workforce to enhance the quality of care (Dixon-Woods, 2019) within a context of:

- increasingly complex population health needs;
- greater demand for health services;
- financial, workforce and other external constraints.

Raising awareness of quality improvement and training healthcare staff in improvement methods has enabled all clinicians to engage in Improvement Science using techniques like the MFI because it addresses an array of quality-of-care issues without the need for advanced training (Silver et al, 2016). The degree of progress, and particularly the evidence that improvement efforts result in actual improvement in the quality of healthcare is, however, limited. Therefore, a major priority for the future is evidencing which improvements are effective and for whom, as well as how improvement is best achieved (Dixon-Woods, 2019). This is particularly important for improvements in patient safety. Despite the impetus resulting from the landmark To Err Is Human Report (IOM, 1999) and developments in the UK such as the introduction of the Concordat for Human Factors in Healthcare (National Quality Board, 2013), much more work is needed. This includes consistently and more effectively translating concepts such as systems science and Human Factors Engineering principles into the design of safer healthcare systems, processes and environments (Bates and Singh, 2018). Crucially, quality improvement needs to become more than an 'artisan activity' (Dixon-Woods, 2019). Addressing concerns about the variable fidelity of QI methods, i.e. the degree to which they are implemented as intended (Dixon-Woods and Martin, 2016), requires more effective Improvement Science education and application, plus the development of Improvement Science role models who are leading the way in nursing.

Activity 7.1   Critical thinking

Re-read Florence's story at the start of Part 3 of this book and consider:

- Was the Charge Nurse that Florence mentioned working with a positive role model for quality improvement or not? What led you to this conclusion?
- How do you think working with this senior nurse influenced Florence's attitude to quality improvement and her potential contribution to this? What evidence led you to this conclusion?

Jot down your answers and discuss with your practice assessor or colleagues. How do their views match or deviate from yours? Why do you think this might be?

Activity 7.1 highlights the importance of role models and context in quality improvement, a topic that is discussed further in Chapter 8. This is important because the contextual and person-centred evidence produced from quality improvement corresponds with the pragmatic, action-orientated and person-centred nature of nursing. This has the potential, however, to become a double-edged sword. This is because the **'production pressure'** of, for example, constantly increasing demand for health services and emphasis on meeting challenging service targets, can drive staff to focus narrowly on the task at hand rather than thinking strategically by considering issues that are out-side their immediate environment but relevant to local improvement efforts. To most effectively use Improvement Science to generate the best context-appropriate evidence and prevent unnecessary repetition, practitioners need to develop a broad, inter-national perspective on improvement (for further details see Busse, 2019 and WHO Sustainable Development Goals for universal health in the additional resources at the end of this chapter).

Future priorities

Quality improvement is a developing discipline and while the practice of qual-ity improvement is increasingly widespread, Improvement Science and empirical evidence, exploring the process of improvement, its effectiveness and impact, is relatively underdeveloped (Dixon-Woods, 2019). This is particularly evident when compared to related academic disciplines like Implementation Science and is a cur-rent criticism of quality improvement. Addressing this challenge is therefore a priority for the future.

Much of the emphasis on quality improvement to date has focused on the practice of continuous quality improvement, often involving small-scale, iterative local improve-ments. A strength of this approach is its proximity to care delivery, as it is based on using the knowledge of clinical staff to identify changes that are predicted to lead to improvement (Silver et al, 2016) and enables knowledge to be generated by local health populations for the issues they view as significant (Clarke and Wilcoxon, 2002). While together these small changes can lead to broader service transforma-tion, this approach is not unanimously viewed as positive, leading to calls for a more strategic and evidence-based approach to improvement (Dixon-Woods, 2019).

Understandably, busy practitioners also tend to focus more on making change without necessarily paying enough attention to establishing the baseline and using robust eval-uation to assess the impact of change against this. As we saw in Chapter 6, however, this is imperative, to determine whether any improvement, no matter how obvious it might seem, is worthwhile; and perhaps more importantly, does not inadvertently make things worse. Previous chapters illustrate that the improvement process is com-plex, non-linear, highly contextual and the effective application of the widely used MFI by nurses in practice can be difficult. Relatively speaking, nursing is evidence-based and protocol driven, therefore dealing with the uncertainty and iterative nature of quality improvement may create challenges, particularly when first engaging with improvement as a new concept and set of skills. Similarly, although PDCA resembles the nursing process, the widespread use of standardised care plans as a way of manag-ing care quality can stifle the development and application of creativity and critical thinking that is necessary for quality improvement in practice. In addition, novice practitioners can be wary of the research and evaluation methods used in improvement work.

Nurses strive to uphold the Code (NMC, 2018b) by keeping their knowledge and practice current and continuously improving on both an individual level and with colleagues. This approach is clearly supported by reflective practice and research, through constant problem-solving with patients and other staff. In fact, the nursing process itself is a problem-solving model that produces pragmatic evaluative evidence to guide practice that is highly contextualised to a specific person and setting. Practitioners like Raj, who we heard from at the start of this chapter, can find it difficult to determine where reflecting on and taking action to improve practice as part of their everyday role using Improvement Science, as is required by the NMC Code (2018b) and the Knowledge and Skills Framework (DH, 2004), ends, and improvement research begins. This is particularly so because in the United Kingdom, for example, students can be required to secure approval for their quality improvement activity using university and healthcare organisation-based governance systems that are primarily designed for research. While both Improvement Science practice and improvement research involve evidencing how best to create and embed improvements in practice to achieve benefits for individuals, teams, organisations and systems, requirements regarding how they are conducted, the type of evidence generated and their wider generalisability differ.

Thus, it can be argued that, while nursing education has enabled staff to effectively link reflective practice and change/theory, advancing this to include Improvement Science in practice by, for example, a greater emphasis on understanding when and how to use Improvement Science and/or improvement research or Implementation Science is a pressing priority.

The global shock created by the Covid-19 pandemic, which was unprecedented in living memory, resulted in many nurse-led service innovations in response. As the recovery continues, it provides a major opportunity for quality improvement to help shape 'the new normal'. This may involve working out how to maintain or adapt service improvements that were prompted by the pandemic and to preserve the improvements achieved, rather than necessarily resorting to pre-pandemic service models. For example, out of necessity the pandemic drove the rapid acceleration of the digitisation of healthcare services. This illustrated great potential benefits as well as pitfalls for stakeholders at all levels from people using services, staff and health organisations, including at country and global levels. Strategic level action plans in development by, for example, WHO Europe and for England (DHSC, 2022), identify improvement opportunities related to this specific issue and Figure 7.1 identifies further examples of priority areas for the application of Improvement Science to address.

- creating fairer, inclusive systems to address health inequalities
- developing more sustainable healthcare systems and integrated services
- enabling better partnership working with service users/carers and other stakeholders, for example to improve safety
- supporting exhausted staff and addressing workforce shortages
- making healthcare more 'doable' or realistic, to enhance safety and workforce wellbeing, for example by the '**de-implementation**' of routine healthcare tasks that are of limited value
- more effectively learning from excellence and **positive deviance**
- wider application and adaptation of Human Factors science to support healthcare improvement

Figure 7.1   Priority areas for the application of Improvement Science

Activity 7.2   Reflection

Reflect on the improvement priorities identified in Figure 7.1 and think about Florence's desired career as a community nurse.

Consider:

1. How might the priorities identified be relevant to community nurses?
2. What other improvement priorities are there in relation to community nursing?
3. What improvement initiatives are planned or already under way in community care that Florence might benefit from being aware of or developing her knowledge of in preparation for her upcoming interview?
4. What might Florence bring as a nurse that adds potential value to the MDT?

If you prefer, complete this activity based on your own field of practice or setting.

When undertaking this activity, you may find it helpful to speak to colleagues and to review your professional body website, community healthcare policy documents or national resources such as NHS Improvement (see the further reading section at the end of this chapter) or equivalent.

Whatever the focus of an improvement topic is, there is a need to move from concentrating on improving healthcare to improving health, by evidencing that improvements to systems, processes and service delivery truly result in better health outcomes for the relevant population.

Nurses as quality improvers within a multidisciplinary team

Nurses and midwives represent the largest group of healthcare professionals and account for approximately 90% of all contacts between patients and healthcare professionals (WHO, 2021b). Year after year nurses are ranked as the most trusted profession in countries around the world; therefore as individuals and a profession they are well-positioned to make a substantial contribution to the continuing improvement of healthcare delivery. In providing a central point of contact, continuity and support for people accessing services and their carers throughout the healthcare journey, the nursing role is recognised – including by other multidisciplinary team members (Cook et al, 2019) – as the glue that holds the team together. Nurses are not always good, however, at recognising their contribution or publicising how this enhances services and improves health outcomes. Time after time the voice of nursing has not been heard or is not even present at the strategic decision-making level for key healthcare policy decisions. The United Kingdom is fortunate to have established national nursing roles such as the Chief Nurse at the Department of Health for each home nation. Though this is still not the case for countries across the globe, efforts to remedy this are ongoing, including for example the recent appointment of a Nursing and Midwifery Policy Advisor for the WHO Europe Region. The shift needed overall, however, will require staff working at all levels of organisations to play their part to ensure the contribution of nurses and nursing to improving the quality of healthcare as members of the multidisciplinary team is acknowledged. To achieve this, nurses must understand how their role as professional citizens relates to the broader improvement context.

Activity 7.3   Building knowledge

Your role as a professional citizen was discussed in Chapter 2. Review your responses to Activities 2.5 and 2.6 to remind yourself of local and organisational examples of how nurses contribute to improving services.

Then, using the information in this chapter, broaden your understanding of the contribution you can make at a strategic level to enhance the future contribution of nursing to improving the quality of care nationally and internationally by:

1. looking at the RCN Foundation Improving Patient Care information to increase your awareness of current improvement priorities for nurses and how to get involved;

(Continued)

(Continued)

2. exploring the International Council of Nurses website and identifying one campaign or way in which they are working to improve the quality of healthcare that is of relevance to you or your area of practice;

3. familiarising yourself with the World Health Organisation's (WHO) Global Strategic Development Goals for achieving universal health coverage, particularly SDG 3 Good Health and Wellbeing, and reflect on how your practice contributes to achieving this wider goal;

4. reading the WHO Global Strategic Directions for Nursing summary. What are the four priority areas? How might what you have learned about improvement be used to support these priorities?

(See the further reading section at the end of this chapter for the four relevant websites.)

Make brief notes on what you have learned from this activity and consider how you might use this knowledge and wider perspective to encourage others to support quality improvement or demonstrate your potential to contribute to improving healthcare outcomes and services to a potential employer.

It is crucial to remember, however, that clinical and other staff are not the only members of the multidisciplinary team (MDT). People accessing services and their advocates must be included as equal partners. To reflect this, they are sometimes referred to as 'honorary members' of the MDT (Edwards, 2002), despite not traditionally being thought of in this way. Their involvement in service level quality improvement efforts is as important as it is for their individual clinical care. This may be achieved formally, through established local or national public involvement groups that have become much more widespread recently, or more informally via local public involvement networks. People accessing services and advocates are key stakeholders; the case study 'Ask the experts' clearly shows how they can provide excellent critical feedback and support for improvement ideas and activity, even when these do not focus directly on them.

Case study   Ask the experts

To free up time for healthcare staff to carry out clinical tasks that were most effective for maintaining patient safety, a team of healthcare practitioners and researchers undertook to identify tasks that clinical staff were required to do but for which the evidence that they enhanced client safety was either non-existent, inconclusive or demonstrated the potential introduction of other safety risks.

Before undertaking a national survey of staff, the team sought views from an established general public/healthcare advocates panel on the overall idea and potential tasks to stop.

While the panel unanimously supported the aim, they suggested the team complete the staff survey first, develop a short-list of potential tasks to be stopped and then consult with public involvement representatives to help determine which task to prioritise stopping and how best to implement this. At that point, the public involvement panel helped identify barriers and facilitators to stopping the task in practice and actively supported the change. This ensured success as their support helped convince clinical staff of the benefits of the change.

Chapter summary

This chapter has considered the current state of quality improvement and nursing's contribution to this agenda. Several important future priorities have been identified, which have been considered in respect of their relevance for the profession, fields of practice and the role of the nurse, as an individual and a member of the multidisciplinary team. The following chapter builds on this by enabling you to consider and plan for the next stage of your development as a quality improver.

Glossary

De-implementation: stopping healthcare practices that add little value to health outcomes and divert staff resources from more beneficial work.

Production pressure: overt or covert organisational pressures and incentives for staff to focus on production, rather than safety, as their primary priority.

Positive deviance: identifying and learning from individuals or groups whose behaviours and strategies are uncommon but result in them finding better solutions to problems than their peers, despite having the same resources and challenges.

Further reading

Busse, R, Klazinga, N, Panteli, D, Quentin, W (Eds) (2019) *Improving healthcare quality in Europe: Characteristics, effectiveness and implementation of different strategies.* Health Policy Series No.53 Brussels: OECD European Observatory on Health Systems and Policies

https://www.icn.ch/ International Council of Nurses

https://www.england.nhs.uk NHS Improvement

https://rcnfoundation.rcn.org.uk/Funded-projects/Improving-Patient-Care RCN Foundation Improving Patient Care

https://www.who.int/publications/i/item/9789240033863 WHO Global Strategic Directions for Nursing

https://www.who.int/health-topics/sustainable-development-goals#tab=tab_117 WHO Sustainable Development Goals– population health and wellbeing goals that all UN Member States have agreed to work towards achieving by the year 2030.

Chapter 8 Quality improvement and you

The future

Gillian Janes and Catherine Delves-Yates

NMC Future Nurse: Standards of Proficiency for Registered Nurses

This chapter will address the following platforms and proficiencies:

Platform 1: Being an accountable professional

1.1 understand and act in accordance with the code: professional standards of practice and behaviour for nurses, midwives and nursing associates, and fulfil all registration requirements.

1.17 take responsibility for continuous self-reflection, seeking and responding to support and feedback to develop their professional knowledge and skills.

Platform 6: Improving safety and quality of care

6.4 demonstrate an understanding of the principles of improvement methodologies, participate in all stages of audit activity and identify appropriate quality improvement strategies.

6.7 understand how the quality and effectiveness of nursing care can be evaluated in practice, and demonstrate how to use service delivery evaluation and audit findings to bring about continuous improvement.

I'm quite confident I have a decent understanding of quality improvement and how to lead improvement in practice now. I know employers are looking for this so I would be able to talk about it at interview, but it all feels a bit woolly when I don't really know where I want to work or what my future focus will be.

(Ali, final year student)

I was frustrated with my lecturer and practice assessor encouraging me to produce a future development plan when, as a student, I wanted to concentrate on passing and getting a job. Their advice was good, however, because at interview I was asked about my development needs and how I could contribute to improving the service I'd be joining. Thinking about these things and developing a plan beforehand meant I was well prepared to answer this, which I'm sure helped me get the job! Also, when my preceptor saw my plan, she helped me connect with improvement specialists in my new workplace.

(Mo, newly qualified nurse)

Introduction

From all the previous chapters you should now have a good understanding of what quality improvement is, why it is relevant for you to develop knowledge and skills in this topic area and how to apply this as part of your everyday nursing role. As we discussed in Chapter 7, there is still plenty of scope for nurses to contribute to quality improvement in practice and a range of priority areas in which you could do so. This chapter will therefore focus on you and your future development as a quality improver by considering how you might continue developing this area of expertise as you prepare for the next phase of your career.

To help you do this we will start by hearing from Harry and Elisabeth, who you met earlier in the book, as they update you on their progress.

Case study   Harry

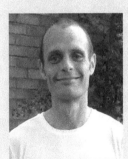

Hello again! We first met in Part 1 of the book, at the start of my nursing programme, when I realised we could improve how patient data was presented in the bedside folders. This change could save time but, more importantly, improve patient safety by reducing the chance of important information being missed. With help from my supervisor and matron the change was tested and adapted using the Model for Improvement as a guide; we got the folders organised effectively with staff happily using them routinely. It worked so well that other areas in the organisation adopted this change too – such a positive outcome!

I am now in my final year and looking back, this was such a good experience. When we were implementing the change, I completed a self-assessment of my improvement capability using the six Cs framework (see Chapter 2). Reviewing this now shows me how much my capability has increased. I still have the same strengths: my ability to care, be compassionate and communicate effectively, although if I could, I would score myself '4' for these now! But the area where I have developed most is courage – to do the right thing for those I care for, to speak up when I have concerns and to have the personal strength and vision to innovate and embrace new ways of working. To me this is the most important of the six Cs and relates directly to being 'an improver' in nursing practice.

Every day I can enhance the quality of the service people receive. I now have the courage, supported by my developing improvement knowledge and experience, to do this. I am currently developing a plan to improve the information people receive about the food they are served in hospital, identifying not only the choices they can make but also the nutritional value. This is the final piece of academic work for my degree, and I aim to implement it in my new role as a Staff Nurse – when I spoke about it at interview, they thought it was a great idea. I still have lots to learn and plenty of work to do but being able to improve things is so motivating!

Case study   Elisabeth

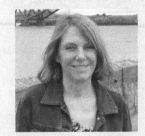

Hello! It's Elisabeth! We first met in Part 2 of the book, when I was at the end of my second year of the nursing programme. I wanted to improve nurse communication during handover. This was the focus of my final piece of academic work and when I got my first staff nurse job, I worked with other members of the team to implement the use of the SBARD tool during handover in our department. While I was really pleased with the grade I got in my degree for the quality improvement plan I wrote, implementing it in practice taught me so much more. To share our experience, we wrote an article that was published and next month we are presenting what we did at a national conference!

The most important thing I learned is that we can always improve care. The conference presentation will discuss what we have done to enhance the change we implemented, as we are continuously improving it – handover can be even better! I never thought I would have the confidence or skills to do this, but when I think about the people we care for and how they deserve best care, it spurs me on! We all need to constantly improve and talking with others helps them to improve their practice too. This experience hugely developed my improvement knowledge and confidence to involve others in trying out new things. This is so important for the delivery of good care and as nurses we are in an ideal position to do it.

Developing knowledge of other improvement strategies

In this book we focus specifically on using just one of many improvement methodologies, i.e. the Model for Improvement (MFI) (Langley et al, 2009), to guide you from start to finish through the process of identifying and leading an improvement in practice as part of your everyday nursing role. We deliberately chose this approach because it helps to focus on a limited range of information when learning something new. This should enable you to develop a solid foundation from which to build expertise and prevent yourself becoming overwhelmed. Chapter 1 introduces the MFI – so if you want to refresh your memory you can review that section before proceeding. Having developed your understanding of the MFI, a commonly used, relatively simple approach to improvement, does not mean you should stop there; you will find, and may already be aware of, other improvement techniques that your organisation uses or that you have heard colleagues talking about. The next step therefore is to familiarise yourself with other commonly used improvement approaches to extend your improvement knowledge and skills and ability to apply these when working in different contexts. Activity 8.1 will help you do this.

Activity 8.1 Building knowledge

Compare and contrast three improvement techniques (apart from the MFI) that are used in healthcare. (If you need examples consider: LEAN, Kaizen (Continuous Improvement), Six Sigma, Total Quality Management (TQM), Business Process Management)

For each technique you have chosen:

(Continued)

(Continued)

- What are the basic principles or elements of the approach?
- Where did the approach originate? I.e. in which sector? When? What could be the implications of this for its application/adaptation in healthcare?
- How has the method been used to improve healthcare services? What examples of application can you find?
- What evidence is there of any benefit or impact from the application of this approach in healthcare?

In addition, talk to colleagues about other improvement approaches they have used or seen used. Doing this demonstrates to others that you value and have an interest in improving services and helps develop your own expertise. See also BMJ Open Quality in the further reading section at the end of this chapter for more examples.

The range of tools that can be used to support the process of improvement we discussed in previous chapters is only a sample of the many available. We have focused on those used most by students and frontline practitioners in healthcare. However, you are highly likely to read about or come across other, equally relevant improvement tools being used in practice. These experiences provide good opportunities to continue developing your understanding of a much wider variety of techniques than an introductory text like this can cover and is therefore encouraged. For example, you may wish to focus more on behavioural science, in which case referring to the Yorkshire Contributory Factors Framework (Lawton et al, 2012) when analysing an issue during Stage 1 of the MFI, or Nudge theory (Thaler and Sunstein, 2008) when designing an intervention, may be particularly useful. Activity 8.2 provides guidance on how to expand your knowledge of different improvement tools but remember, this process is an ongoing journey and you will add to your improvement skillset throughout your career.

Activity 8.2   Building knowledge

Make a list of the quality improvement tools you have learned about or tried out in previous chapters, then review the toolkit resources in Chapter 4 (further reading section) and Quality Improvement Essentials Toolkit – Institute for Healthcare Improvement (IHI) (register for a free account to access these resources if you haven't previously done so).

Focusing specifically on tools you are not familiar with:

- Choose 2–3 and make brief notes in your own glossary of terms that you were encouraged to develop in the Introduction chapter.
- Speak to colleagues with improvement experience about the new tools you have listed – what experience of them do they have, when have they seen them used, how and to what effect etc.?

Communicating your quality improvement capability to others

Communicating your capability to others, including potential employers, requires self-awareness and healthy self-esteem or self-worth. At this point it would be useful to remind yourself of where you were at the start of this book by reviewing the results of the self-assessments you undertook in Chapter 2 to enhance your self-awareness of your initial leadership and improvement capability. In addition, review your notes from Activity 5.1 in Chapter 5, where you considered what had stimulated your idea for improvement and how this helped you to fulfil the requirements of the NMC Code (2018b) and the 'Future Nurse' proficiencies (NMC 2018a).

Nurses are renowned for not publicising their achievements or contribution to care. As we saw in Chapter 7, it is sometimes colleagues, other members of the MDT, that more readily recognise these. Learning to share your talents and successes in a natural way without coming across as arrogant does not necessarily come easily to even the most accomplished of people and yet is a key personal leadership skill in the modern world (Klaus, 2004). We may all like to think that doing excellent work is enough to spread good practice or support your own career; however, as is also highlighted in Chapter 6, this is not necessarily so. One of the difficulties many nurses have in recognising their own contribution can be linked to the term 'expert'. For example, when do you become an expert? If this resonates personally it might help to think about it in terms of 'gravitas'. Gravitas can be thought of as the ability to command trust and respect from others and Goyder (2014) uses the following equation to represent how multiple components come together to create this characteristic in an individual:

Gravitas = Knowledge + Purpose + Passion − Anxiety

Using this equation to frame how you think about your expertise and contribution to improvement can be helpful in overcoming the 'imposter syndrome' felt by many practitioners. Ensure that you identify aspects of improvement knowledge and skills you wish to enhance, then if you have some trepidation about taking the next step in your career, this will be balanced by a clear purpose as well as your passion for ensuring people receive the best care possible. The increased recognition of the value of clinical knowledge and skills to the systematic and evidence-based enhancement of practice, for example in the form of clinical academic roles and joint clinical/university appointments, which are now becoming more widespread, should also help. This may be a pathway you want to consider in your future career plan, but first, Florence who we met at the start of Part 3 of this book has an update for us.

Case study   Florence

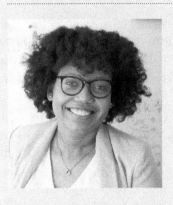

Hi! It's Florence! I shared my story in Part 3 of the book, but I want to add my thoughts about the skills we bring from our previous work and life experiences – 'transferrable skills' – that also help equip us to improve care.

As nurses we are often not good at identifying our own expertise, either for personal development or to share with others. We do, however, all have a wide range of skills and competencies we use every day to navigate daily life. We are all leaders, leading ourselves and others such as our family, friends and professionally, where we frequently apply leadership skills when working with others in our nursing role. For example, I have two young children and caring for them has developed my organisational and communication skills greatly; I must plan and negotiate with others to ensure my children are looked after so I can attend placement or study during 'out of school' hours. I first applied and developed these skills as a Health Care Assistant, then almost every day since I started the nursing programme; and being involved in improvement gives me the opportunity to enhance these skills further.

So don't forget what you do outside the nursing programme and any professional care roles you have. If you think about what you do just to get yourself to placement or university on time, run your home and have food in the cupboard, I am sure you will identify other transferrable skills you can use for improving healthcare too!

Take the first step of assessing your current improvement capability by completing Activity 8.3; it focuses on a new job but you could adapt it to consider a new placement or in preparation for your next personal development review.

Activity 8.3   Reflection

Review a job description for your next role, looking specifically at the quality improvement-related criteria. Make notes on how you could demonstrate your ability against these based on your knowledge and experience of the topic to date. Some things to think about as you do this are:

- Which past experiences or achievements could you use to demonstrate your ability and/or potential against these criteria?
- Which aspects of these achievements might it be relevant to highlight? e.g. how you involved the relevant stakeholders, which improvement methodology/change theory/leadership skills did you use? How did you maintain and evaluate progress?

- Which transferable skills do you have that could be applied to the improvement aspects of this role? For example, when have you had to convince others to support you in making change? (don't forget any roles you have held outside nursing.)

Discuss your conclusions from this reflection with your lecturer, practice supervisor or a trusted friend/colleague. Ask them to help you identify any illustrative or transferable examples you might have missed.

Reviewing your progress and forward planning

Lifelong learning is expected of all healthcare professionals and demonstrating your ongoing development is a formal requirement of continuing professional registration through the revalidation process. Continuing professional development is relevant to all aspects of the NMC Code (2018b), but of specific interest here are two main areas, i.e. Practise Effectively and Preserve Safety. Similarly, all the Future Nurse proficiencies platforms are related to the nurse's role in quality improvement although this is most predominantly the case for platforms 1 (Being an accountable professional), 5 (Leading and managing nursing care and working in teams), 6 (Improving safety and quality of care) and 7 (Co-ordinating care). Having completed the activities and learning in this book, now is a good time to develop a plan for the next stage of your progress as a quality improver based on a review of how far you have come.

Activity 8.4 Measuring

Review the self-assessment you undertook in Chapter 2 regarding your personal and technical improvement knowledge and skills and the action plan you developed to enhance these. Reflect on and make a note of the elements in the plan you have achieved and the general progress you have made in developing your improvement expertise.

Next review your response to Activity 8.3 – which areas were you finding it difficult to demonstrate experience of, and for which ones could you only give limited responses or examples?

Based on these reflections and focusing on how your quality improvement knowledge and skills have changed, revise your personal action plan from Chapter 2 or draft a new one to guide your further improvement skills development over the next 1–2 years. You may find it helpful to refer to the Conceptual Model of Improvement (see Foundations chapter Figure F1) to remind yourself of the different components of Improvement Science when doing this activity.

We encourage you to complete this activity in discussion with your practice assessor; you may also find it useful to seek advice from a colleague with quality improvement experience or by talking to an improvement practitioner in your organisation.

Considering the need for nursing role models in quality improvement discussed in Chapter 7, we suggest you consider how you might demonstrate good quality improvement practice to others as you go about your everyday work. Identifying the support you need to do this and how you could access or generate this will be time well spent.

Adopting a staged approach to your development as a quality improver is likely to be most productive. For example, what will be your priorities for the next three, six, 12 and 24 months? Also, what aspirations do you have that either depend on your achievement of these short-term goals or will take longer to achieve? – these could be your longer-term goals/priorities. This is a very individual process that will be influenced by many factors including, for example, how far into the nursing programme you are when you start this process, local organisational context and your previous life and work experiences.

You may wish to become the 'go to person' for quality improvement in your team – or ultimately the whole organisation – but need to gain more experience of being involved in improvements in practice or learn about new improvement techniques to enable you to achieve this longer-term goal. Although the focus here is on further developing your quality improvement expertise, take Florence's advice from earlier and do not forget your transferable skills, i.e. leadership, communication, person-centred care focus, empathy or assertiveness, for example, as these can also be developed simultaneously, enabling your broader personal development as a qualified practitioner and leader in the profession.

In terms of transferable learning, do not limit yourself to the traditional application of tools that you are familiar with or be afraid of thinking differently. For example, Figure 8.1 demonstrates how one of the authors applied their knowledge of quality improvement to support reflection on and communication of their career and contribution to healthcare through applying the MFI in a creative and novel way.

Chapter summary

This chapter has encouraged and enabled you to review how your improvement knowledge, skills and competency have changed as a result of your learning and suggests how to develop a practical plan for enhancing these further. This included the creative and novel application of the explanatory MFI to support reflection on your personal development. The work you have undertaken in the activities in the previous chapters places you in an excellent position from which to continue improving person-centred care services in collaboration with patients, carers and other members of the multidisciplinary team.

Hopefully you will have found this textbook helpful in supporting the development of your quality improvement expertise and contribution. We wish you every success as you move forward.

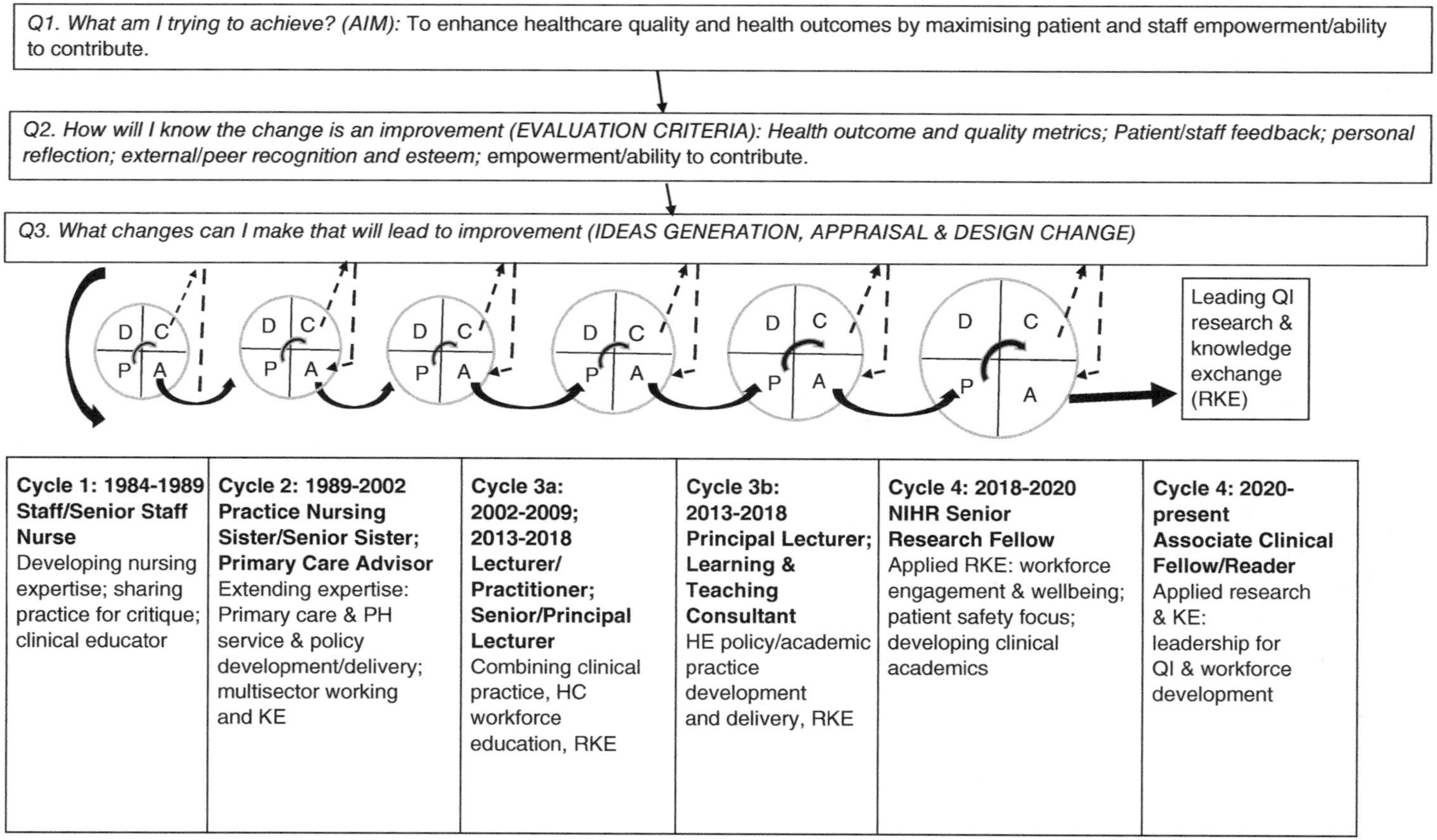

Q1. What am I trying to achieve? (AIM): To enhance healthcare quality and health outcomes by maximising patient and staff empowerment/ability to contribute.

Q2. How will I know the change is an improvement (EVALUATION CRITERIA): Health outcome and quality metrics;; Patient/staff feedback; personal reflection; external/peer recognition and esteem; empowerment/ability to contribute.

Q3. What changes can I make that will lead to improvement (IDEAS GENERATION, APPRAISAL & DESIGN CHANGE)

Leading QI research & knowledge exchange (RKE)

Cycle 1: 1984-1989 Staff/Senior Staff Nurse Developing nursing expertise; sharing practice for critique; clinical educator	Cycle 2: 1989-2002 Practice Nursing Sister/Senior Sister; Primary Care Advisor Extending expertise: Primary care & PH service & policy development/delivery; multisector working and KE	Cycle 3a: 2002-2009; 2013-2018 Lecturer/ Practitioner; Senior/Principal Lecturer Combining clinical practice, HC workforce education, RKE	Cycle 3b: 2013-2018 Principal Lecturer; Learning & Teaching Consultant HE policy/academic practice development and delivery, RKE	Cycle 4: 2018-2020 NIHR Senior Research Fellow Applied RKE: workforce engagement & wellbeing; patient safety focus; developing clinical academics	Cycle 4: 2020-present Associate Clinical Fellow/Reader Applied research & KE: leadership for QI & workforce development

PH – Public Health, KE –Knowledge Exchange, RKE – Research and Knowledge Exchange, HC – Healthcare

Figure 8.1 Application of explanatory MFI: integrating and applying the art and science of leadership for quality improvement to improve health outcomes

Useful websites

https://bmjopenquality.bmj.com/ BMJ Open Quality – open access journal publishing case study reports of improvement in practice.

http://www.ihi.org/education/IHIOpenSchool/Chapters/Pages/default.aspx Information on Institute for Healthcare Improvement chapters network

https://q.health.org.uk/ Quality Improvement Network – access to peer support and resources – apply for free membership when you are able to demonstrate you have led successful improvement on a wider scale than your own team.

References

Alderwick, H, Charles, A, Jones, B and Warburton, W (2017) *Making the Case for Quality Improvement: Lessons for NHS Boards and Leaders.* London: The Kings Fund.

Alderwick, H and Ham, C (2017) Sustainability and transformation plans for the NHS in England: what do they say and what happens next? *British Medical Journal*, 356: j1541.

Atkinson, S, Ingham, J, Cheshire, M and Went, S (2010) Defining quality and quality improvement. *Clinical Medicine*, 10 (6): 537–9.

Auerbach, AD, Landefeld, CS and Shojania, KG (2007) The tension between needing to improve care and knowing how to do it. *The New England Journal of Medicine*, 357 (6): 608.

Baily, MA, Bottrell, M, Lynn, J and Jennings, B (2006) *The Ethics of Using QI Methods to Improve Health Care Quality and Safety: A Special Report.* New York: The Hastings Centre.

Bansal, S. (n.d.) How to create a Gantt chart in Excel – Batman style. *Available online at:* https://trumpexcel.com/gantt-chart-in-excel/ (accessed 12 July 2022).

Bates, DW and Singh, H (2018) Two decades since To Err Is Human: an assessment of progress and emerging priorities in patient safety. *Health Affairs*, 37 (11): 1736–43.

Bennis, W (1989) *On Becoming a Leader.* London: Random House.

Bridges, W (1991) *Managing Transition: Embracing Life's Most Difficult Moments.* Cambridge, MA: Pereus Publishing.

Bridges, W (1986) Managing organizational transitions. *Organizational Dynamics*, 15 (1): 24–33.

Busse, R, Klazinga, N, Panteli, D and Quentin, W (eds) (2019) *Improving Healthcare Quality in Europe: Characteristics, Effectiveness and Implementation of Different Strategies.* Health Policy Series No.53. Brussels: OECD European Observatory on Health Systems and Policies.

Card, AJ (2017) The problem with '5 whys'. *BMJ Quality and Safety*, 26: 671–7.

Carter, H (2017) How to write a robust business case for service development. *Nursing Times*, 113 (7): 25–8.

Chin, R and Benne, K (1985) General strategies for effecting changes in human systems, in Bennis W, Benne K and Chin R (eds) *The Planning of Change* (4th edn). New York: Holt, Rinehart & Winston.

Cialdini, R (2009) *The Psychology of Influence and Persuasion.* New York: Harper Collins e-books. Available online at: https://learning.oreilly.com/library/view/influence/9780061899874/text/9780061899874_Cover.xhtml (accessed 10 June 2022).

CIEHF (2019) *Human Factors and Healthcare Evidencing the Impact of Human Factors Training to Support Improvements in Patient Safety and to Contribute to Cultural Change.* Wootton Wawen: Chartered Institute of Ergonomics and Human Factors.

Clark, R and Kemp, W (2008) Using the six principles of influence to increase student involvement in professional organisations; a relationship marketing approach. *Journal of Advanced Marketing Education,* 12: 46.

Clarke, CL and Wilcockson, J (2002) Seeing need and developing care: exploring knowledge for and from practice. *International Journal of Nursing Studies,* 39: 397–406.

Collins *English Dictionary* (2021). Available online at: https://www.collinsdictionary.com/dictionary/english/mindset (accessed 12 July 2022).

Collins, B (2018) *Adoption and Spread of Innovation in the NHS.* London: The Kings Fund.

Cook, O, McIntyre, M, Recoche, K and Lee, S (2019) 'Our nurse is the glue for our team': Multidisciplinary members' experiences and perceptions of the gynaecological oncology specialist nurse role. *European Journal of Oncology Nursing,* 41: 7–15.

Cribb, A, Entwistle, V and Mitchell, P (2020) What does 'quality' add? Towards an ethics of healthcare improvement. *Journal of Medical Ethics,* 46: 118–22.

Connelly, L. M. (2021) Using the PDSA model correctly. *Medsurg Nursing,* 30 (1): 54–61.

Davidoff, F and Batalden, P (2005) Toward stronger evidence on quality improvement. Draft publication guidelines: the beginning of a consensus project. *BMJ Quality and Safety,* 14 (5): 319–25.

Delves-Yates, C (2021) *Beginner's Guide to Reflective Practice in Nursing.* London: Sage.

Department of Health (DH) (2012) *Compassion in Practice: Nursing, Midwifery and Care Staff: Our Vision and Strategy.* London: HMSO.

DH (2009) *The NHS Constitution.* London: Crown Copyright.

DH (2004) *Simplified Knowledge and Skills Framework (KSF).* London: NHS Employers. Available online at: https://www.nhsemployers.org/SimplifiedKSF (accessed 12 July 2022).

DHSC (2022) *A Plan for Digital Health and Social Care.* London: GOV.UK. Available online at: www.gov.uk (accessed 9 July 2022).

Dixon, N (2017) *Guide to Managing Ethical Issues in Quality Improvement or Clinical Audit Projects.* London: Healthcare Quality Improvement Partnership.

Dixon, N (2021) *Guide to Managing Ethical Issues in Quality Improvement or Clinical Audit Projects.* London: Healthcare Quality Improvement Partnership.

Dixon-Woods, M (2019) How to improve healthcare improvement: an essay by Mary Dixon-Woods. *British Medical Journal,* 366: 15514.

Dixon-Woods, M and Martin, GP (2016) Does quality improvement improve quality? *Future Hospital Journal,* 3 (3): 191.

Dixon-Woods, M, McNicol, S and Martin, G (2012) Ten challenges in improving quality in healthcare: lessons from the Health Foundation's programme evaluations and relevant literature. *BMJ Quality & Safety,* 21 (10): 876–84.

Donabedian, A (2005) Evaluating the quality of medical care. *The Milbank Quarterly*, 83 (4): 691–729.

Eby, K (2021) *The Essential Guide to PDSA*. Available online at: https://www.smartsheet.com/content/plan-do-study-act-guide (accessed 13 July 2022).

Edwards, C (2002) A proposal that patients be considered honorary members of the healthcare team. *Journal of Clinical Nursing*, 11 (3): 340–8.

EKR Foundation (2022) Kubler-Ross change curve. Available online at: https://www.ekrfoundation.org/5-stages-of-grief/change-curve/ (accessed 9 July 2022).

Ellis, P (2019) *Leadership, Management and Team Working in Nursing*. London: Sage.

Fisher, J (2012) *Process of Personal Transition*. Available online at: https://www.r10.global/wp-content/uploads/2017/05/fisher-transition-curve-2012-1.pdf (accessed 4 April 2022).

Flodgren, G, Hall, AM, Goulding, L, Eccles, MP, Grimshaw, JM, Leng, GC and Shepperd, S (2016) Tools developed and disseminated by guideline producers to promote the uptake of their guidelines. *Cochrane Database of Systematic Reviews*, 8. Available online at https://pubmed.ncbi.nlm.nih.gov/27546228/ (accessed 17 August 2022).

Francis, R (2013) *Report of the Mid Staffordshire NHS Foundation Trust Public Inquiry*. London: Crown Copyright.

Fulton, JS (2019) Professional citizenship. *Clinical Nurse Specialist*, 33 (4): 153–4.

Glouberman, S and Zimmerman, BJ (2002) *Complicated and Complex Systems: What Would Successful Reform of Medicare Look Like?* Discussion paper #8 Commission on the Future of Health Care in Canada. July. Available online at http://change-ability.ca/Health_Care_Commission_DP8.pdf (accessed 17 August 2022).

Goyder, C (2014) *Gravitas: Communicate with Confidence, Influence and Authority*. London: Vermillion.

Grimshaw, J, Eccles, M, Thomas, R, MacLennan, G, Ramsay, C, Fraser, C and Vale, L (2006) Toward evidence-based quality improvement. *Journal of General Internal Medicine*, 21 (2): S14.

Gronn, P. (2000) Distributed properties: a new architecture for leadership. *Educational Management & Administration*, 28(3): 317–38.

Ham, C, Berwick, D and Dixon, J (2016) *Improving Quality in the English NHS: A Strategy for Action*. London: The Kings Fund.

Ham, C, Alderwick, H, Dunn, P and McKenna, H (2017) *Delivering Sustainability and Transformation Plans: From Ambitious Proposals to Credible Plans*. London: The Kings Fund.

Health Europa (2019) One in ten NHS Trusts are fully digitised, despite plans for a paperless NHS. Available online at: https://www.healtheuropa.eu/paperless-nhs-2/91746/ (accessed 25 June 2022).

Healthcare Improvement Scotland (2017) *Handy Guide to Measurement for Improvement*. Glasgow: Healthcare Improvement Scotland.

Heslop, P, Blair, P, Fleming, P, Hoghton, M, Marriott, A and Russ, L (2013) *Confidential Inquiry into Premature Deaths of People with Learning Disabilities (CIPOLD)*. Bristol: Norah Fry Research Centre.

Hewitt-Taylor, J (2013) *Understanding and Managing Change in Healthcare: A Step-By-Step Guide.* London: Palgrave Macmillan. Available online at: https://ebookcentral.proquest.com/lib/uea/reader.action?docID=4008025# (accessed 28 June 2022).

Holland, JH (1992) *Adaptation in Natural and Artificial Systems: An Introductory Analysis with Applications to Biology, Control, and Artificial Intelligence.* Cambridge, MA: MIT Press.

HQIP (2017) *Patient and Public Involvement in Quality Improvement.* London: HQIP. Available online at: https://www.hqip.org.uk/wp-content/uploads/2019/05/Nov-2017-update-HQIP-PPI-in-QI-Guide.pdf (accessed 12 July 2022).

Iacobucci, G (2020) Plan to digitise NHS will fall short without extra investment, says spending watchdog. *British Medical Journal* (Clinical Research edn), 369, m1972. https://doi.org/10.1136/bmj.m1972

IHI (2022) *Science of Improvement.* Institute for Healthcare Improvement. Available online at: http://www.ihi.org/about/Pages/ScienceofImprovement.aspx (accessed 1 April 2022).

Institute of Medicine (IOM) (2001) *Crossing the Quality Chasm: A New Health System for the 21st Century.* Washington DC: National Academy Press.

IOM (1999) *To Err Is Human: Building a Safer Health System.* Washington DC: Institute of Medicine.

Jabbal, J (2017) *Embedding a culture of improvement.* London: The Kings Fund.

James, KT (2011) *Leadership in Context: Lessons from New Leadership Theory and Current Leadership Development Practice.* London: The Kings Fund.

Janes, G, Harrison, R, Johnson, J, Simms-Ellis, R, Mills, T and Lawton, R (2022) Multiple meanings of resilience: health professionals' experiences of a dual element training intervention designed to help them prepare for coping with error. *Journal of Evaluation in Practice*, 28 (2): 315–23.

Klaus, P (2004) *Brag!: The Art of Tooting Your Own Horn without Blowing It.* New York: Grand Central Publishing.

Kotter, JP (2012) *Leading Change.* Boston: Harvard Business Review Press.

Landsberg, M (2003) *The Tools of Leadership.* London: Profile Books.

Langley, GL, Moen, R, Nolan, TW, Norman, CL and Provost, LP (2009) *The Improvement Guide: A Practical Approach to Enhancing Organizational Performance* (2nd edn). San Francisco: Jossey-Bass.

Lawton, R, McEachan, RRC, Giles, SJ, Sirriyeh, R, Watt, IS and Wright, J (2012) Development of an evidence-based framework of factors contributing to patient safety incidents in hospital settings: a systematic review. *BMJ Quality and Safety*, 21: e369–e380.

Lewin, K (1951) *Field Theory in Social Science.* New York: Harper.

Leybourne, SA (2016) Emotionally sustainable change: two frameworks to assist with transition. *International Journal of Strategic Change Management*, 7 (1): 23–42.

Locock, L, Parkin, S, Montgomery, C and Chisholm, A (2021) How frontline teams engage with patient-centred quality improvement. *Nursing Times*, 117 (2): 34–36.

Available online at https://www.nursingtimes.net/clinical-archive/patient-experience/how-frontline-teams-engage-with-patient-centred-quality-improvement-18-01-2021/ (accessed 17 August 2022).

Lucas, B and Nacer, H (2015) *The Habits of an Improver*. London: The Health Foundation.

MacDonald, M (2020) *The Health and Social Care Workforce Gap*. London: Crown. Available online at: https://commonslibrary.parliament.uk/the-health-and-social-care-workforce-gap/ (accessed 12 July 2022).

Mach, M, Abrantes, ACM and Soler, C (2021) Teamwork in healthcare management, in Firstenberg, MS and Stawicki, SP (eds) *Teamwork in Healthcare* (pp. 347–470). London: Intechopen.

Mager, RF (1997) *Preparing Instructional Objectives: A Critical Tool in the Development of Effective Instruction* (3rd edn). Atlanta, GA: Center for Effective Performance.

Maher, L, Gustafson, D and Evans, A (2010) *Sustainability Model and Guide*. Coventry: NHS Institute for Innovation and Improvement.

Martin, GP, Sutton, E, Willars, J and Dixon-Woods, M (2013) Frameworks for change in healthcare organisations: A formative evaluation of the NHS Change Model. *Health Service Management Research*, 26 (2–3): 65–75.

Miller, D (2001) Successful change leaders: What makes them? What do they do that is different? *Journal of Change Management*, 2 (4): 359–68.

Moldovan, F (2020) Framework specifications for evaluation of quality improvement and sustainable development in healthcare facilities. *Proceedings*, 63 (1): 2.

Molloy, A, Martin, S, Gardner, T and Leatherman, S (2016) *A Clear Road Ahead: Creating a Coherent Quality Strategy for the English NHS*. London: The Health Foundation.

Montgomery, C, Parkin, S, Chisholm, A and Locock, L (2020) 'Team capital' in quality improvement teams: findings from an ethnographic study of front-line quality improvement in the NHS. *BMJ Open Quality*, 9: e000948.

Mortimer, F, Isherwood, J, Wilkinson, A and Vaux, E (2018) Sustainability in quality improvement: redefining value. *Future Healthcare Journal*, 5 (2): 88–93.

Murad, M. H. (2017, March). Clinical practice guidelines: a primer on development and dissemination. In *Mayo Clinic Proceedings*, 92 (3): 423–33. Elsevier.

National Quality Board (2013) *Human Factors in Healthcare: A Concordat from the National Quality Board*. London: NHS England.

NHS England (2014) *Five Year Forward View*. NHS England. Available online at https://www.england.nhs.uk/wp-content/uploads/2014/10/5yfv-web.pdf (accessed 12 July 2022).

NHS England (2016) *Leading Change, Adding Value: A Framework for Nursing, Midwifery and Care Staff*. London: NHS England.

NHS England (2017) *The Fifteen Steps Challenge*. London: NHS England.

NHS England (2018) *The Change Model Guide*. London: NHS England. Available online at: https://www.england.nhs.uk/wp-content/uploads/2018/04/change-model-guide-v5.pdf (accessed 27 January 2022).

NHS England (2019) *The NHS Long Term Plan.* London: NHS. Available online at: www.longtermplan.nhs.uk/publication/nhs-long-term-plan (accessed 4 April 2022).

NHS England (2021) *QSIR – Plan Do Study Act.* Available online at https://www.england.nhs.uk/wp-content/uploads/2021/03/qsir-plan-do-study-act.pdf (accessed 27 January 2022).

NHS England and Improvement (2018) *Quality, Service Improvement and Re-design Tools: A model for measuring quality care.* Available online at: https://www.england.nhs.uk/wp-content/uploads/2022/02/qsir-measuring-quality-care.pdf (accessed 12 July 2022).

NHS England and NHS Improvement (n.d.) *Online Library of Quality, Service Improvement and Redesign Tools: Seven Steps to Measurement for Improvement.* London: NHS England/NHS Improvement. Available online at: https://www.england.nhs.uk/wp-content/uploads/2021/12/qsir-seven-steps-to-measurement-for-improvement.pdf (accessed 12 July 2022).

NHS England and NHS Improvement (2022) *Plan, Do, Study, Act (PDSA) Cycles and the Model for Improvement.* London: NHS England and NHS Improvement. Available online at https://www.england.nhs.uk/wp-content/uploads/2022/01/qsir-pdsa-cycles-model-for-improvement.pdf (accessed 17 August 2022).

NHS Improvement (2016) *Developing People – Improving Care: A National Improvement and Leadership Framework for the NHS.* London: NHS Improvement. Available online at https://eoe.leadershipacademy.nhs.uk/wp-content/uploads/sites/6/2019/04/10591-NHS_-Improving_Care-Summary.pdf (accessed 17 August 2022).

NHS Improving Quality (2014) *First Steps towards Quality Improvement: A Simple Guide to Improving Services,* available at: https://bit.ly/3NqDyvA (accessed 07 September 2022)

NHS Institute for Innovation and Improvement (2005) *Improvement Leaders' Guide: Evaluating Improvement.* Coventry. Available online at https://www.england.nhs.uk/improvement-hub/publication/improvement-leaders-guide-evaluating-improvement-general-improvement-skills/ (accessed 17 August 2022).

NHS Institute for Innovation and Improvement (2010) *Sustainability Model and Guide.* Available online at https://www.england.nhs.uk/improvement-hub/wp-content/uploads/sites/44/2017/11/NHS-Sustainability-Model-2010.pdf (accessed 17 August 2022).

NHS Institute for Innovation and Improvement (2010) *The Handbook of Quality and Service Improvement Tools.* West Midlands: New Audience Ltd.

NHS Leadership Academy (2013) *Healthcare Leadership Model.* Leeds: NHS Leadership Academy.

Nicolini, D, Waring, J and Mengis, J (2011) Policy and practice in the use of root cause analysis to investigate clinical adverse events: Mind the gap. *Social Science & Medicine,* 73 (2): 217–25.

NMC (2015) *Guidance on Using Social Media Responsibly.* London: Nursing and Midwifery Council.

NMC (2018a) *Future Nurse: Standards Framework for Nursing and Midwifery Education (SFNME).* London: Nursing and Midwifery Council.

NMC (2018b) *The Code: Professional Standards of Practice and Behaviour for Nurses, Midwives and Nursing Associates.* London: Nursing and Midwifery Council.

National Survivor User Network (NSUN) (2015) *Nothing Without Us.* London: NSUN.

Ockenden, D (2022) *Findings, Conclusions and Essential Actions from the Independent Review of Maternity Services at The Shrewsbury and Telford Hospitals NHS Trust.* London: Crown.

Ogrinc, G, Davies, L, Goodman, D, Batalden, PB, Davidoff, F and Stevens, D (2016) SQUIRE 2.0 (*Standards for QUality Improvement Reporting Excellence*): Revised publication guidelines from a detailed consensus process. *BMJ Quality and Safety*, 12: 986–92.

Orlando, I (1961) *The Dynamic Nurse–Patient Relationship.* New York: Putnam.

Oxlade, L (2020) *The Courage of Compassion: Supporting Nurses and Midwives to Deliver High-Quality Care.* London: The King's Fund. Available online at https://policycommons.net/artifacts/1715937/the-courage-of-compassion/2447552/ (accessed 17 August 2022).

Parkin, P (2009) *Managing Change in Healthcare: Using Action Research.* London: Sage. Available online at: https://ebookcentral.proquest.com/lib/UEA/detail.action?Docid=635500 (accessed 28 June 2022).

Penning, J (1975) Interdependence and complementarity: the case of a brokerage office. *Human Relations*, 28 (9): 825–40.

Penny, J (2003) *Improvement Leaders Guide: Improvement Knowledge and Skills.* London: NHS Institute for Innovation and Improvement.

Perigo, G and Callaghan, S (2011) *Commissioning for Outcomes: A Resource Guide for Commissioners of Health and Social Care.* Oxford: NHS Oxford Health. Available online at: https://www.oxfordhealth.nhs.uk/library/news/commissioning-for-outcomes-a-resource-guide-for-commissioners-of-health-and-social-care/ (accessed 12 July 2022).

Plesk, P (2003) *Complexity and the Adoption of Innovation in Health Care.* Washington DC: National Institute for Health Care Management Foundation/National Committee for Quality Health Care.

RCN (2021) *Nursing Workforce Standards: Supporting a Safe and Effective Nursing Workforce.* London: Royal College of Nursing.

Reed, JE and Card, AJ (2016) The problem with plan-do-study-act cycles. *BMJ Quality & Safety*, 25 (3): 147–52.

Rooke, N and Phipps, J (2022) Becoming a change agent, in Delves-Yates, C (ed.) *Essentials for Nursing Practice* (3rd edn, Chapter 9). London: Sage.

Rowland, P, McMillian, S, Martimianakis, MA and Hodges, BD (2018) Learning from patients: constructions of knowledge and legitimacy in hospital-based quality improvement programmes. *Studies in Continuing Education*, 40 (3): 337–50.

SCIE (2015) *Co-production in Social Care: What It Is and How to Do It – at a Glance.* London: Social Care Institute for Excellence.

Sebok-Syer, SS, Shaw, JM, Asghar, F, Panza, M, Syer, MD and Lingard, L (2021) A scoping review of approaches for measuring 'interdependent' collaborative performances. *Medical Education*, 55 (10): 112–30.

Sfantou, DF, Laliotis, A, Patelarou, AE, Sifaki-Pistolla, D, Matalliotakis, M and Patelarou, E (2017, December) Importance of leadership style towards quality of care measures in healthcare settings: a systematic review. *Healthcare*, 5 (4): 73, Multidisciplinary Digital Publishing Institute.

Sheingold, BH and Hahn, JA (2014) The history of healthcare quality: the first 100 years 1860–1960. *International Journal of Africa Nursing Studies*, 1: 18–22.

Silver, SA, Harel, Z, McQuillan, R, Weizman, AV, Thomas, A, Chertow, GM, Nesrallah, G, Bell, CM et al. (2016) How to begin a quality improvement project. *Clinical Journal of the American Society of Nephrol*, 11 (5): 893–900.

Sloan, L and Quan-Haase, A (eds) (2017). *The SAGE Handbook of Social Media Research Methods*. London: Sage.

Tabak, RG, Khoong, EC, Chambers, DA and Brownson, RC (2012) Bridging research and practice: models for dissemination and implementation research. *American Journal of Preventive Medicine*, 43 (3): 337–50.

Taylor, MJ, McNicholas, C, Nicolay, C, Darzi, A, Bell, D and Reed, JE (2014) Systematic review of the application of the plan–do–study–act method to improve quality in healthcare. *BMJ Quality & Safety*, 23 (4): 290–8.

Thaler, H and Sunstein, CR (2008) *Nudge*. London: Penguin.

The Health Foundation (2011) *Evidence Scan: Improvement Science*. London: The Health Foundation.

The Health Foundation (2015) *Evaluations: What to Consider Commonly Asked Questions about How to Approach Evaluation of Quality Improvement in Healthcare*. Available online at: https://www.health.org.uk/publications/evaluation-what-to-consider (accessed December 2021).

The Health Foundation (2021) *Quality Improvement Made Simple: What Everyone Should Know about Health Care Quality Improvement*. London: The Health Foundation. Available online at: www.health.org.uk/publications/quality-improvement-made-simple (accessed 17 August 2022).

Thompson, JD (1967) *Organisations in Action: Social Science Bases of Administrative Theory*. New York: McGraw-Hill.

Van Emden, J and Becker, L (2016) *Presentation Skills for Students*. Basingstoke: Palgrave. Available online at: https://ebookcentral.proquest.com/lib/UEA/detail.action?docID=6234930 (accessed 27 June 2022).

Vigier, M and Bryant, M (2009) The astonishment report: a pedagogical tool to assist students in learning from their international experience. *Global Business Languages*, 14 (5). Available online at: http://docs.lib.purdue.edu/gbl/vol14/iss1/5 (accessed 8 August 2022).

Wageman, R (1995) Interdependence and group effectiveness. *Administrative Science Quarterly*, 40 (1): 145–80.

Weaver, P (2007) *The origins of modern project management*. Paper presented at the Fourth Annual PMI College of Scheduling Conference. Available online at https://www.

mosaicprojects.com.au/PDF_Papers/P050_Origins_of_Modern_PM.pdf (accessed 17 August 2022).

West, M, Collins, B, Eckert, R and Chowla, R (2017). *Caring to Change: How Compassionate Leadership Can Stimulate Innovation in Health Care.* London: The King's Fund.

West, M, Eckert, R, Steward, K and Pasmore, B (2014) *Developing Collective Leadership for Health Care.* London: The Kings Fund.

West, MA (2021) *Compassionate Leadership: Sustaining Wisdom, Humanity and Presence in Health and Social Care.* London: Swirling Leaf Press.

WHO (2021a) *Innovation.* Available online at: https://www.who.int/topics/innovation/en/ (accessed 24 January 2021).

WHO (2021b) *Global Strategic Directions for Nursing and Midwifery 2021–2025.* Geneva: World Health Organization.

Wilson, PM, Petticrew, M, Calnan, MW and Nazareth, I (2010) Disseminating research findings: what should researchers do? A systematic scoping review of conceptual frameworks. *Implementation Science,* 5 (1): 1–16.

Wolcott, MD, McLaughlin, JE, Hann, A, Miklavec, A, Beck-Dallaghan, GL, Rhoney, DH and Zomorodi, M (2020) A review to characterise and map the growth mindset theory in health professions education. *Medical Education in Review,* 55 (4): 430–40.

Wong, KC, Woo, KZ and Woo, KH (2016) Ishikawa diagram, in O'Donohue, W and Maragakis, A (eds) *Quality Improvement in Behavioral Health.* Cham, Switzerland: Springer.

Wyatt Knowlton, L and Phillips, C (2013) *The Logic Model Guidebook: Better Strategies for Great Results.* London: Sage.

Index

Note: References in *italics* are to figures, those in **bold** to tables; 'g' refers to key terms.

Printed in the USA
CPSIA information can be obtained
at www.ICGtesting.com
CBHW071910110624
9876CB00004B/33

9 781529 768978